Neris and India's
Idiot-Proof Diet
How we lost ten stone

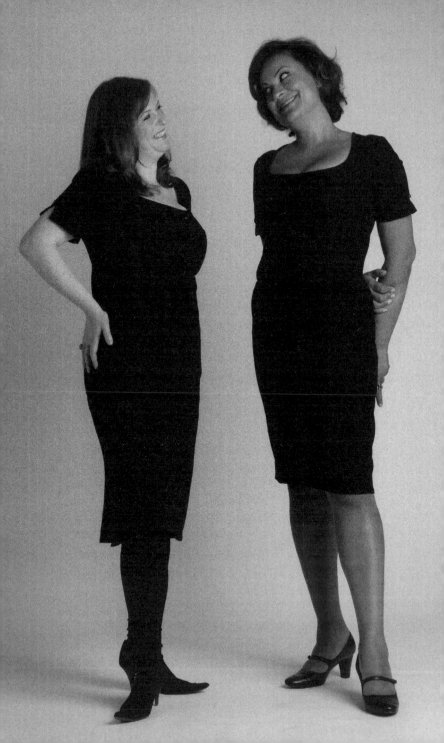

Neris and India's Idiot-Proof Diet

How we lost ten stone

India Knight and Neris Thomas

who would really like to call this book

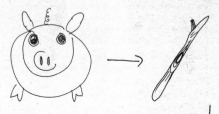

FROM PIG TO TWIG !

Illustrations by Neris Thomas

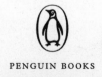

PENGUIN BOOKS

PENGUIN BOOKS

Published by the Penguin Group
Penguin Books Ltd, 80 Strand, London WC2R ORL, England
Penguin Group (USA) Inc., 375 Hudson Street, New York,
    New York 10014, USA
Penguin Group (Canada), 90 Eglinton Avenue East, Suite 700, Toronto,
    Ontario, Canada M4P 2Y3 (a division of Pearson Penguin Canada Inc.)
Penguin Ireland, 25 St Stephen's Green, Dublin 2, Ireland (a division of
    Penguin Books Ltd)
Penguin Group (Australia), 250 Camberwell Road, Camberwell,
    Victoria 3124, Australia (a division of Pearson Australia Group Pty Ltd)
Penguin Books India Pvt Ltd, 11 Community Centre, Panchsheel Park,
    New Delhi - 110 017, India
Penguin Group (NZ), 67 Apollo Drive, Rosedale, North Shore 0632,
    New Zealand (a division of Pearson New Zealand Ltd)
Penguin Books (South Africa) (Pty) Ltd, 24 Sturdee Avenue, Rosebank,
    Johannesburg 2196, South Africa

Penguin Books Ltd, Registered Offices: 80 Strand,
    London WC2R ORL, England

www.penguin.com

First published by Fig Tree 2007
Published with an Afterword in Penguin Books 2008

Copyright © Neris Thomas and India Knight, 2007, 2008

3

Illustrations copyright © Neris Thomas, 2007
Photographs copyright © Shaun Webb, Neris Thomas and India Knight, 2007

The moral right of the authors has been asserted

Designed and typeset by Smith & Gilmour, London
Set in Plantin and Thesis Sans
Colour reproduction by Dot Gradations Ltd, UK
Printed in Great Britain by Clays Ltd, St Ives plc

A CIP catalogue record for this book is available from the British Library

ISBN: 978-0-141-02743-2

**This diet is not suitable for pregnant or nursing women, children,
diabetics or people with kidney disease. It is not entirely impossible
to follow if you are vegetarian, but it is not by any means vegetarian-
friendly. Always consult your doctor before embarking on a new eating
plan. If you are diabetic, we very highly recommend Dr Richard K.
Bernstein's *The Diabetes Diet***

www.greenpenguin.co.uk

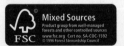

Mixed Sources
Product group from well-managed
forests and other controlled sources
www.fsc.org Cert no. SA-COC-1592
© 1996 Forest Stewardship Council

FSC

Penguin Books is committed to a sustainable future
for our business, our readers and our planet.
The book in your hands is made from paper
certified by the Forest Stewardship Council.

Contents

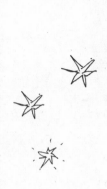

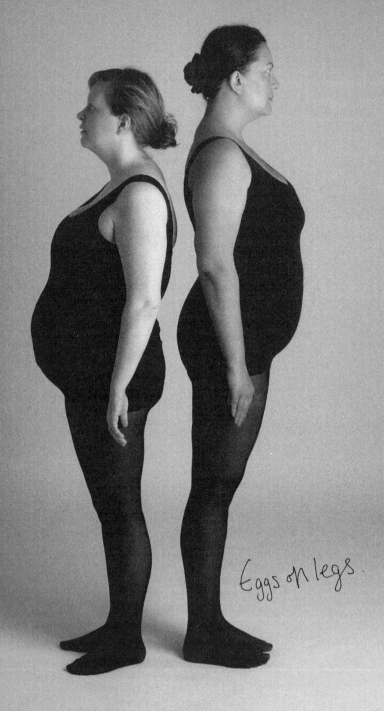

Eggs on legs.

Introduction

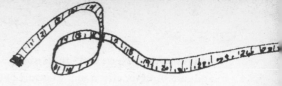

So here we have it: yet another diet book. And none of the usual qualifications for writing one, either – we're not doctors, we're not nutritionists, we're not former soap stars on our uppers. We're not unusually obsessed by other people's poos, happily enough. We have no immediate plans for an exercise DVD.

Ho no. We can do better than that.

Between us, Neris and I have lost ten stone, give or take the odd pound. It took us a year, and we have maintained the weight loss. Ten stone is a lot of weight. It's a shedload. It's as much as a whole other person (Lordy, what a thought). And we think it's pretty damned impressive. Unusual, too. Show us a diet book written by someone who's actually lost more than a few measly pounds and we'll eat a whole bag of potatoes and a tub of lard for seconds. Other diet book writers talk the talk. We walk the walk. Well, we walk it now. We used to just waddle, thighs chafing attractively together.

That's the problem with the usual diet books. We're not going to say they don't work, because many of them do – the majority, probably – why wouldn't they? All kinds of diets work; the problem is sticking to them. That's because diet books are not written by people with a lot of weight to lose. They don't come from the minds of the formerly fat. So you get these grim, gloomy volumes of finger-wagging directions: boil a fish, steam a sprout, run for two hours. And those books are unbelievably depressing. They make you feel like you've been punished, excluded from normal life, and they make you want to give up before you've even begun. They expect you to do ridiculous things, and eat in a ridiculous way – one that, we've found, is not sustainable in the long term, and that is of itself incredibly demoralizing. Most diets are a disaster if you have families; they sit there with their delicious dinner, you sit there nibbling on a leaf, feeling leprous. It's just horrible.

We really like food – this diet was conceived and developed

in a restaurant. Neris and I used to meet for lunch every week and one summer afternoon, a couple of bottles in, we got to talking about weight, for the hundredth time. Neris had just bought *The GI Diet* and could make neither head nor tail of it; India – as you will read in a minute – had had a moment of extreme sartorial crisis in a department store. We both knew we needed to lose weight and suddenly, during our conversation, the idea became a real possibility – because it occurred to us that we could do it together. Two minds are better than one, after all, and we liked (rightly, it turns out) the idea of the inbuilt support system.

We're greedy, which is how we came to be so weeble-ish in the first place. And while we understood, when we first embarked on our diet, that we would obviously have to make *some* sacrifices, we didn't want to feel like total freaks, either. We wanted to be able to go out for dinner. We wanted to eat at friends' houses without first having to email them a great, long, tiresomely anti-social list of our dietary requirements. We wanted to go to the pub, on girls' nights out, to weddings, to parties, and not feel like Fatty On a Diet sitting in the corner with a diet soda and a crudité.

We all know what to do to lose weight, in theory: eat less and move around more just about covers it. Makes sense. Sounds perfectly reasonable. Indeed, it *is* perfectly reasonable, if you want to lose five pounds. But the eat-less/move-more method is a thin person's mantra, and comes from a thin person's mindset. If you're the kind of person that weighs eight stone and occasionally 'forgets to eat', eat-less/move-more is blindingly obvious and true. But we've never forgotten to eat – in fact, we used to be starving hungry at pretty much any given time of the day. We don't have a thin person's mindset, one that assumes the self-discipline that many dieters – ourselves included – find easy to grasp in theory but rather trickier to put into practice. For us, eat-less/move-more simply isn't enough. Nice idea, but some people are just, well, *too fat* for such a vague instruction.

Besides, eat-less/move-more doesn't even begin to address what goes on in your head when it comes to food, or the fact that so much overeating is emotional. And it fails to acknowledge that the gym is anathema if you're uncomfortable with the concept of crop tops, bare arms and paying for the pleasure of being in a room full of toned, trim people who are your physical opposites. If it were really as simple as eating a wee bit less and doing more sit-ups, we'd all be waifs.

What we wanted was to find a way of eating that was on the one hand very straightforward – no calorie-counting, no points, no having to think too hard – and on the other incredibly detailed. We wanted a plan to adhere to. A serious plan that went into minute detail, but that was flexible. Not a fortnight's worth, either; we wanted precise directions to stick to for as long as it took – which is why this book gives you a lifetime's worth of instructions. And we wanted recipes that we'd want to cook regardless of whether or not we were on a diet (and cheaty, easy-peasy recipes for when we didn't feel like cooking). We wanted to know what to eat and drink in any number of situations, at any given time of day – including feeling a bit peckish at midnight, or weirdly ravenous at 11am – so that we never had to pause to ask ourselves what was and what wasn't allowed. It feels very comforting, sticking to a plan in this way, and sooner or later you learn it by heart and it becomes second nature. And it absolutely, 100 per cent hand-on-heart works: check out the pictures for the rather hideously graphic evidence.

Is it easy? Kind of. We're going to start this book as we mean to go on, which means absolutely no lies (it works both ways: we don't want you to lie to yourself any more either – much more on this later). For the majority of the time, it's so easy that you completely forget you're on a diet. Sometimes it's harder. Very occasionally, you'll feel pretty majorly pissed off, to be frank. But the elation you feel as the pounds drop off and the compliments start flowing should override any difficulties, and besides, you're going to be eating delicious food – warm, hearty, rib-sticking food of the kind that is not usually associated with the word 'diet'. We're not expecting you to survive on salad. Our way of eating is not going to interfere with your life, either. It just quietly goes on in the background while you get on with the other stuff, such as selling your too-big clothes on eBay once a month. In terms of easiness, the thing we found vitally important about our diet was to understand that in order for it to work, the transformation – the moment when it all clicks into place – needs to happen before you start out, not after. That means right now. There will, obviously, be a dramatic physical transformation at the end of your diet, but we have discovered that for any diet to succeed, an emotional transformation is not only necessary but crucial. That means starting off at a place of self-love, not self-disgust. It means making the most of yourself right now – not tomorrow, not in a month, not in a year's time. We know you're beautiful now (and we're going to be showing you ways of building on that) – but we need you to believe it too. In our now considerable experience, no diet will work long term until that 'mental click'. It is a powerful and invaluable tool. If you have no idea of what we're talking about here, read on: the first part of the book is all about getting you to the point where you have faith in yourself.

We're working mothers, with four children between us. We have babies, jobs, dogs, partners, houses to clean, chores to do, homework to supervise, stuff going on. We don't have the time to cook ourselves separate meals, or to avoid the supermarket for fear of temptation, or to work out for a couple of hours a day. Life is short, and we are busy. And yet, almost miraculously, we've dropped all this horrible weight (and yes, it was horrible. Horrible, horrible, horrible[1]) without much hardship. We thought we'd tell you how we did it.

We make no spectacular claims for the diet; like we said above, all sorts of diets work. We chose to go the low-carb route. There is no earth-shattering hype to the way we dieted, no magic trick, except 1: it works – and how; 2: it allows you

[1] For more on the myth of the Happy Fatty, see page 22.

to live a normal life; and 3: crucially, you don't feel deprived, punished, denied, or like you're sitting in the corner wearing a big Fatty hat.

Neris and I were lucky – we did the diet together, which was like having your own mini support system. This book is here to fulfil the same function: think of it not just as a manual but as your friend, there by your side through thick and thin, through success and failure, through the bad days as well as the good ones. Carry it in your handbag. Re-read it often. Scribble in it and make notes. Let the recipe pages get sticky with use. Learn to love it – and yourself. It won't let you down.

Before that, though, let's go back to the beginning. How did we get so bloody fat in the first place? Do try to read this next bit, and not skip straight to the actual diet, because we have found that understanding how and why we got fat really helped us to understand how and why to stay thin, or thinner. That's another thing: we're not body-fascists. We don't believe that everyone should be a size ten (or, God forbid, a size oo). By all means, go ahead and shrink to a ten if that's what you really want, but please understand that there's a cut-off point. If you started off being a size twenty-two, for instance, you may find yourself blissfully, deliriously happy being a size sixteen. Remember that, a: you need to set yourself realistic goals, because crazily unrealistic goals are the ones that are easiest to abandon; and b: there comes a stage in weight-loss when your face goes all wrinkly and gaunt, like a very old monkey's, and in our book it's a stage best avoided. Wrinkly and gaunt is not a good look on anyone. Also, grim things can happen to your boobs, if you go from vast to minute. More on this in the relevant chapter, but please bear it in mind. You want to look fabulous – and more often than not, that means curvy, not anorexic. This is especially true if you're anywhere upwards of forty, because if you want to keep wrinkles at bay and generally look well, rather than gaunt or slightly simian, you have to be careful not to get too skinny. There's a lot of truth in the saying that, past forty, you need to choose between your arse and your face. We say it's a no-brainer: go for the face, every time. Unless you work in the adult film industry and earn your living as somebody's arse-double, obviously.

Here's a table, in good old feet, inches and pounds, which can help you determine a healthy and foxy-looking weight for your height and build.

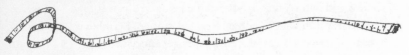

Height	Small Frame	Medium Frame	Large Frame
4'10"	102–111	109–121	118–131
4'11"	103–113	111–123	120–134
5'0"	104–115	113–126	122–137
5'1"	106–118	115–129	125–140
5'2"	108–121	118–132	128–143
5'3"	111–124	121–135	131–147
5'4"	114–127	124–138	134–151
5'5"	117–130	127–141	137–155
5'6"	120–133	130–144	140–159
5'7"	123–136	133–147	143–163
5'8"	126–139	136–150	146–167
5'9"	129–142	139–153	149–170
5'10"	132–145	142–156	152–173
5'11"	135–148	145–159	155–176
6'0"	138–151	148–162	158–179

So, the podge. How did it get there? How did we get to the point where we became experts at avoiding communal changing rooms, at never acknowledging a full-length mirror, at flicking past the fashion pages of magazines because not a lot of clothes came in our size, at never having sex on top (excess flesh + gravity = aargh)? It's a long story, but worth telling, we think, because chances are yours is pretty similar.

The Stakes

We found it helpful to know precisely why weight loss was so important to us – the 'why here, why now?' question. We also found it helpful to keep reminding ourselves of these stakes, at various stages of the diet – it helps focus the mind. These were our stakes as we began the diet. Please fill in yours, and refer back to them whenever you're feeling wobbly or doubtful.

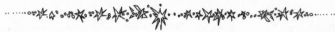

Neris:

▸ I wanted to get back to pre-pregnancy weight.
▸ I wanted to buy clothes in a normal shop.
▸ I wanted to be at my sister-in-law's wedding and look and feel good.
▸ I wanted to stop crying hysterically at transformation programmes on telly.
▸ I wanted to feel that my husband fancied me.
▸ I wanted my wedding ring to fit me again.
▸ I wanted to wear the size fourteen jacket I bought six years ago.
▸ I wanted to be fit, for my daughter's sake.

India:

▸ I wanted to go shopping and be able to buy any clothes from any shop.
▸ I wanted to wear high heels and not feel they might snap.
▸ I wanted to feel physically confident enough to be naked.
▸ I wanted my children to feel proud of the way I looked.
▸ I wanted to buy bracelets that fitted my wrists.
▸ I wanted to stop feeling foggy and lethargic.
▸ I wanted to look nice in photographs.
▸ I wanted to look hot for my fortieth birthday party.

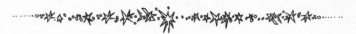

What are your initial stakes?

Write them down here.

_____

_____

_____

_____

_____

_____

_____

_____

_____

_____

_____

_____

_____

_____

_____

_____

_____

_____

_____

_____

_____

_____

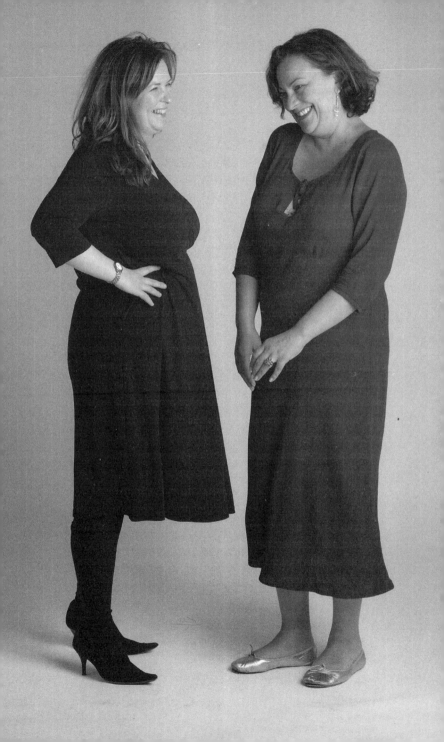

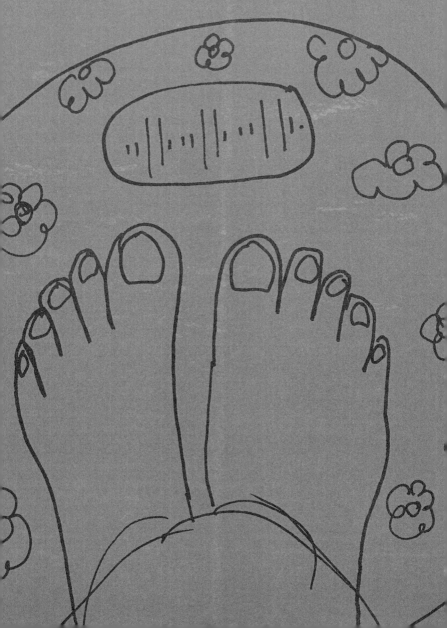

1. Our Diet Histories

India

I was never fat. I was a tall, skinny child – flat-chested, no hips
to speak of, very often mistaken for a boy. I always liked food –
I come from a family that really appreciates their dinners – but
I also regarded it as fuel. It appeared three times a day, I ate it,
I ran off to play.

I went to boarding school at thirteen which, looking back,
is where I think the problem started. The seeds of it were
sown, at any rate. My mother is a fantastic cook, as were all the
women in my family, and I was brought up eating really well
in several different countries. My previous (day) school had
been French, and its lunches were, as far as I can remember,
pretty nice. Now I suddenly found myself in the depths of
Buckinghamshire, faced with old-school-style meals I simply
couldn't eat. It's the usual story: boiled mince, grey and worm-
like, overcooked vegetables and weird, fatty, gristly bits of meat
that looked and tasted like donkey. No spices, no dressings, no
flavour at all, as far as I was concerned. And it all smelled vile.
We were supposed to finish everything on our plates, because
of the starving children in Africa. I was always having to stay
behind with my housemistress, while she sat hectoring me, and
I mutinously refused to eat, and she told me I had to, for hours
on end. I actually threw up a couple of times, once while being
forced to eat stuffed lambs' hearts. I don't want to sound too
princess-and-the-peaish about this, but it really was difficult:
the food we were given literally stuck in my throat. And,
obviously, being at boarding school, this went on for weeks and
weeks at a time – I couldn't run home and have a nice supper at
the end of the day.

I eventually realized that I liked puddings. I don't have a
sweet tooth, oddly enough (my downfall is salty things, like
cheese and biscuits), but those very English things like steamed
sponge and custard, or spotted dick, or jam roly-poly did at
least taste quite nice. The breakfasts were okay, too – I ignored

the congealed, lumpy porridge and filled up on toast (plastic bread) with extra butter. We had a gas fire in the common room, and we used to sneak out bread, butter and Marmite and make toasties. We were allowed out into the local town on Saturday mornings, and stocked up on crisps and sweets and, in my case, Ritz crackers and cheese biscuits. Parents could come and take us out to tea, which someone or other's did most Saturdays, and I'd be taken along as a guest and encouraged to devour the full monty, with scones and clotted cream and tiers of little cakes and sandwiches (The Copper Kettle in Marlow still holds a special place in my heart). When no parents materialized, the school provided a fairly fancy tea anyway, every day. More bread, more cakes, more stodge.

At this point, my incredibly carb-heavy diet wasn't a problem: we walked for miles every day and games were compulsory. Much as I loathed them at the time, they saved me from being completely spherical. But, a: I learned to associate food with comfort – the toasties and cakes and Double Deckers from the tuck shop acting as respite from the grey weariness of school life, food generally being something nice to turn to whenever I felt lonely or bored; and b: I developed a life-long love of, and dependence on, carbohydrates. Which, as we will see, are the devil when they are totally processed, bleached and fiddled about with until they are shorn of any goodness or nutritional value.

I left boarding school at seventeen, when I was a size twelve to fourteen on top (I have big tits) and a ten underneath. I'm five feet ten, so this seemed about right. I lived at home some of the time, or in flats with girlfriends, and food didn't really feature much – I was too busy running about having a lovely time. I ate a lot of cereal (more carbs) and a lot of sandwiches (ditto), usually at weird times of the day.

At eighteen I went to university. While the food in college was marginally better than the food at school – along the same lines, though – I more or less dispensed with it and cooked for myself. I was a student, I didn't have much money, and I basically lived on pasta for three years. Oh, and chips. And pitta bread and hummus. And then, of course, there was alcohol – rivers of it. We drank all the time, as though it was perfectly normal, which maybe for students it is. It is also unbelievably fattening, at least if your mixer of choice is lemonade, as mine was, and your favourite drink is (or was) Southern Comfort. At this point, needless to say, the daily walks and the compulsory lacrosse had gone out the window, though I did bicycle everywhere. I left university a size fourteen to sixteen on top and a twelve below. I was well upholstered, shall we say, more curvaceous than was entirely fashionable, but I looked pretty good, in a 1950s kind of way. I certainly had no 'issues' with my weight. Indeed I never weighed myself: I didn't own a pair of scales until the summer of 2005.

Life went on. I worked in a series of newspaper offices, which are seldom what you'd call dry zones. Pub at lunchtime. Quick drink or three after work. More sandwiches, grabbed on the hoof. Crisps. Sausage rolls. Chocolate bars and biscuits and cups of sugary tea. Egg McMuffins. No more bicycling, exercise down to zero, unless you count walking to and from the Tube. I was a sixteen all over, and it had just started to bother me slightly – I was reconciled to the tits, but the size sixteen waist wasn't part of the plan. I'd got to the stage where I vaguely thought I probably ought to do something about it. Then I got pregnant.

Chances are you've been there. It's so bloody hard to shift, isn't it? And it hardly seemed to be a priority; I was too busy being delighted with my baby to worry too much about my waistline, or the lack of it. But it was at this point, aged around twenty-seven, that I started having minor difficulties with clothes shopping. I could no longer buy anything very fitted or tailored; it just really didn't look good. But I put it to the back of my mind and lived, as many young mothers do, in leggings and baggy jumpers. When I needed to dress up, I wore forgiving, stretchy things with a high Lycra content. I took comfort in the knowledge that I still had good legs; if I felt fat,

I'd wear slightly shorter skirts and a bit of a heel. It didn't occur to me at the time that I was storing all my weight on my upper half, or that I was heading for egg balanced on pipe cleaners territory. I still didn't own a set of scales.

I got pregnant again a few years later, and had a second Caesarean section. By this stage my stomach – never my best feature – was a disaster area. I avoided looking at it in the bath and made sure my then husband never got a look at it. I was so successful at concealing it from him that one year he bought me some Agent Provocateur lingerie for Christmas, complete with tiny, sexy little knickers which, had I worn them, would have sat right on my C-section scar, with my excess of stomach muffining attractively over the top.

The stomach wasn't the only thing muffining. At home all day with two small children, I seemed to be eating constantly. I'd make the boys breakfast, and hoover up their leftovers. We'd have a snack at about eleven. I drank cups and cups of tea, with one big sugar per cup. I'd have my lunch, then pick at theirs. Then I'd pick at their tea. Then I'd make dinner, and eat it with my (irritatingly whip-thin) husband. We'd usually have some wine, and then blob out on the sofa, perhaps with a bag of crisps. I used food as punctuation to my day: when the boys had a nap, I'd have a biscuit. When I'd dropped the eldest off at nursery, I'd have more tea and toast.

I got fatter and fatter – incrementally, not dramatically. What is really weird about this period is that, while I could obviously tell that I was getting bigger, I was oddly reluctant to do anything about it (and this reluctance continued, unbelievably to me now, for *well over a decade*). There are several reasons for this, and I think they're worth examining.

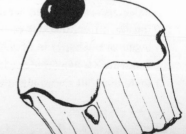

1. Arrogance. There isn't a likeable way of putting this, so I won't bother trying. I thought I was still pretty good-looking. Okay, maybe not first thing in the morning, puffy from lack of sleep and with baby sick on my dressing gown. But I scrubbed up well. You perfect all kinds of tricks when you're unhappy with your weight, and one of mine was makeup. With a face full of artfully applied slap, a pair of control-top knickers, some cleavage on show and a good haircut, I thought I looked all right. More than all right, actually. I'd always been popular; I'd never in my life been short of boyfriends. My husband clearly found me attractive; my trusty bathroom mirror (head and shoulders only) was flatteringly lit; I'd learned never to look down past my bosom; and I could be extremely charming when I felt like it. I behaved like a confident person – indeed I was a confident person, about everything except my weight. My weight bothered me. But not enough to do anything concrete about it. I was pretty cocky. And very complacent.

Oh, and another thing: I'd always had (and still have) a real horror of the kind of women who obsess about their weight. It seemed to me to be deeply uncool. I hated people who called chocolate cake 'sinful', just as I hated those very thin women who push a salad leaf around their plate and call it lunch. If the choice was between being like them and being on the Rubenesque side, there was no contest. It didn't occur to me that there was a middle way.

2. A weird, skewed acceptance of fate. There was a part of me which thought that my youth was over (in my twenties!) and that being slightly overweight was the price you paid for being a married woman with children. I didn't have many friends in the same boat – most of the women I knew who had children were older than me, and had 'let themselves go', as I saw it. I thought this was what you did. I sort of carried my extra weight as a badge of honour: 'I'm no longer the flibbertigibbet you once knew. I am a woman of substance (literally). I have better things to do than faff about with a step machine.' I'd had a pretty good innings, I thought, being young and attractive, and if I carried a bit too much heft, well, hey, there were worse things.

3. Bloody-mindedness. Like the smoker who smokes an extra packet on National Non-Smoking Day, I ate an extra helping every time someone mentioned weight. That someone was pretty much without fail my mother, who only had to mention the phrase 'losing a few pounds' for me to unleash a giant tirade about how she was un-feminist and retrograde, and how women didn't have a wretched duty to be attractive at all times, especially when they were knackered from running around after two small children and at home all day long. 'It's not the 1950s,' I'd mutter crossly, before helping myself to a Danish pastry.

4. Dawn French, I'm sorry to say, and other vocal self-proclaimed Happy Fatties. They were quite persuasive there, for a while. They made a very good job of equating fatness with sensuality, appetite for food with appetite for life, the inability to resist thirds with largeness of spirit. Fat women, they seemed to be saying, loved life, and lived it in a joyous, celebratory way that thin people didn't. I believed this, or more accurately made myself believe it for convenience's sake. I even bought an outfit by French & Teague, which made me look like a beached whale. And then there was all the stuff about men loving curves, much of it written by Vanessa Feltz shortly before her husband dumped her.

This thing about men is just delusional, I'm afraid. Men like a nice rack. Men don't like a flappy pouch of skin overhanging the stomach, or droopy upper arms, or more than one chin. But nobody said this (it would have been 'fattist'), and women all over the place decided it was easier to believe this guff than to go on a diet. I was one of them. And when I thought of myself, it was as Anita Ekberg in *La Dolce Vita*, not – more realistically – as Brutus from *Popeye*.

Another thing about Dawn French: she is very, very pretty. Unusually so. She is perhaps marginally less pretty as a size twenty-six than she would be as a size fourteen, but not much. That's why she looks good: not because she's fat, but *despite* it. This is not a trick many people can pull off. Besides, having a pretty fat face doesn't magically exclude you from the horrendous health risks of being obese. And your body still looks like a doughnut.

5. Laziness, which overlaps with arrogance. This one is self-explanatory. I had no energy – partly because of haring around after the children, but partly (though I didn't know it at the time) because I ate enormous quantities of stupor-inducing food, which totally sapped me of strength. I was permanently exhausted. I felt like a nap within a couple of hours of waking up. So I'd sit at the kitchen table and nibble things instead.

6. (This is a weird one) Deliberately bulking up. Done subconsciously, but over the years I've spoken to dozens of women who say they've done the same thing.

We're now five years on from all of the above. As my marriage started falling apart, I did the very opposite of what you'd expect someone in that situation to do (pine away): I ate more. I didn't, as far as I am aware, do this consciously. But having thought about it, and compared notes with friends, it seems to be true that, in moments of stress, some women bump up the portions to make themselves bigger. Bigger equals stronger, braver, harder to squash, harder to hurt, harder to ignore or dismiss. It's as though the fat becomes a carapace, a sort of protective outer shell which will shield you from harm. Illness, divorce, stress, the death of a parent: if you're the 'coper' in your family (and I always have been), chances are you'll realize at some stressful point that you can't actually cope at all. You don't want to create more stress by admitting this, so you coddle and 'reward' yourself with food, which has the supplementary benefit of making you 'bigger' in all respects – 'My shoulders are broad' – not all of them bad in coping terms. There is certainly an apparent comfort (it's another delusion, but never mind) in feeling you are big enough to take anything life throws at you: it's a 'Come and have a go, if you think you're hard enough,' thing. Easier to say, or feel, this when you're not a scrawny little shrimp. Some women start doing this in childhood.

7. I should probably also mention that a close relative had an eating disorder from the age of fourteen. In my head, weight issues were her department. Some members of my immediate family had a peculiar-seeming relationship with food: irrational hatreds of some random things, an odd take on vegetarianism, a devotion to health food shops, a compulsion to order off-menu. Sometimes they were on the plump side, sometimes they were rakes. My mother either ate a lot or didn't eat at all. I thought of myself as the sensible one when it came to food: I didn't make a fuss and I ate everything. Literally.

I don't want to oversell this by making myself sound like I hit a size thirty-two during this period. I was a size eighteen – sometimes the eighteen was looseish, sometimes it was skin-tight. And then, in the late spring of 2005, my size eighteen clothes suddenly stopped fitting. And that, dear reader, was when I finally decided I'd had enough. It was 15 July at around 2pm. I was in the fat people's department of Selfridges (they don't call it that, of course – they call it something absurd like 'relaxed clothing') and suddenly I felt like bursting into tears. I also felt a great rush of anger – rage, really – at what I'd done to myself. It was a moment of revelation. A light went on in my head, and I thought, 'For fuck's sake. ENOUGH!' 'Scuse my French, but that's what I thought, verbatim.

Unlike Neris, who as we shall see is a champion dieter of many years' standing, I'd never got to this point before. I had, as I've mentioned, a little panoply of tricks – magic knickers, makeup, décolletage, self-deprecating jokes, blah blah blah. I remember feeling murderous at a party some years ago, when a woman – then rather admired for her sartorial style – came up to me and complimented me on mine. 'You're so well dressed,'

she said. 'I love the way you're so comfortable with your size.'
She wasn't being a bitch (I don't think), but I wanted to stab
her. But encounters like this were the exception rather than
the norm. And in my head, until 15 July 2005, I wasn't a carb-
guzzling blimp. I was 'slightly overweight'. That was all.

But as the clouds parted and the dazzling light shone down
to expose the truth, I realized that that wasn't all at all. I WAS
A SIZE TWENTY. I was a woman in my prime, frankly, with
an okay face and a well-proportioned body, and for some crazy
reason known only to myself, I was entering my fortieth year
weighing nearly sixteen stone – the same as two skinny people
welded together. It wasn't okay. It didn't look nice, or even
a little bit nice. It was utterly grotesque. A few times in the
previous couple of months, I'd decided at the last minute not to
attend a party that I'd really been looking forward to. I told my
boyfriend it was because I was tired. I wasn't tired at all. I was
too fat. I had, for the first time ever, become embarrassed to
be seen in public, is the truth of it. I had nothing to wear.
I was Giant bloody Haystacks.

I told myself so many lies. Here are some of them:

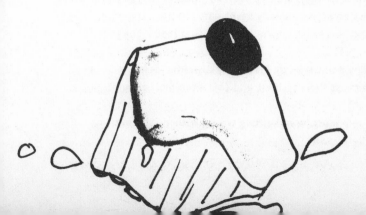

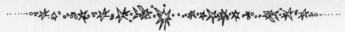

I am curvy, not fat.
As we have seen, this is pure delusion. Curvy people aren't egg-shaped.

Okay. Then I'm Rubenesque. Junoesque. You know, voluptuous.
Those are synonyms of 'fat'. And you're in denial.

I have a bubbly personality.
I don't at all, actually. I developed a personality to match my weight – I turned myself into a jolly fat person because it seemed appropriate. I am much grumpier now I'm thinner, and it suits me just fine. And dropping the self-deprecating fat jokes – 'I'll just insult myself, shall I, before you insult me' – has been heaven.

I am still rather marvellously physically attractive.
Really? To whom – weirdo chubby-chasers? And (horrified gulp) do I want my boyfriend/husband to have people think that he's one of them?

I'm awfully unphotogenic.
No, just really fat. The camera doesn't lie. Not 100 per cent of the time, anyway.

How glad I am not to be a self-obsessed clothes-horse!
Well, it's hard to be, when normal clothes don't fit you.

These knickers are so comfy. Silly little scraps of lace are for sissies, or the sexually desperate.
And how I wish with all my heart that I could buy them.

Why don't M&S do bras in my size? The fools.
Because there's a limit, and 40H is probably about it.

There must be something wrong with my thyroid.
There wasn't.

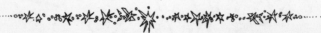

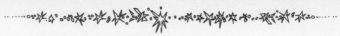

I look good naked. I must feel quite nice.
Then why be scared of full-length mirrors? Why be shy of walking around naked? Why come out of the shower and make a point of never, ever looking down?

I have very wide feet.
No, just fat feet (and I've gone down a shoe size since starting the diet).

I can't see my feet because I have such big tits.
True. Also, such a big stomach.

I have big hands.
No, just fat fingers (and my rings have had to be adjusted since I lost weight).

I'm a fun person. I like to eat, drink and be merry.
Well, I certainly ate and drank. But it made me about as merry as a six-mile tailback. And there's nothing 'fun' about seconds of mash. You don't dole yourself out another scoop, clapping your hands with delight while thinking, 'Wahoo! This is great fun!' Or if you do, you need to get out more.

Ooh, I just love life. I devour it, me.
People who love life don't turn themselves into blimps, risk their health, impair their sex lives, or make it impossible for themselves to ever walk around in their underwear. People who love shopping (and I do, so much so that I wrote a whole book about it) don't exclude themselves from ninety-nine per cent of clothes shops because there's nothing in their size.

At least I'm not some ghastly, neurotic, brittle, anorexic-looking obsessive. Take me out to lunch, and I eat.
True. But the choice isn't between looking like Victoria Beckham or Johnny Vegas. There is a middle way.

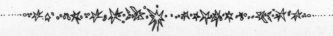

And so on. There were dozens of these lies, as you'll see
– they're scattered throughout the book. Our mission is to
demolish them one by one.

But back to 15 July. There I was, boiling with rage,
surrounded by hideous plus-size (waaah) clothes for outsize
matrons. I put down whatever elasticated-waist horror I'd been
examining and marched down to the basement, to the books
department, where I bought all the diet books I'd ever heard
of. I started reading them that night. The ones that made most
sense were Atkins, South Beach, the Zone, Protein Power and
the GI Diet. South Beach and Atkins have an identical Phase
1, lasting a fortnight. What you are holding in your hands right
now is our take on the above diets: we cherry-picked, and then
made up our own version.

I went to the supermarket the next day, and started dieting
– for the first time in my life – on 17 July.

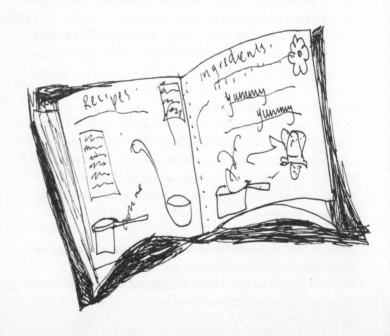

Neris

I've done Slimfast, liver detox and fasting. I've had kinesiology. I've had my blood examined for allergies only to discover I'm allergic to haddock and I don't like haddock anyway. I've had the Zone Diet delivered to my door every day for two months, only to eat the perfectly proportioned food as snacks between meals. I've done colonic irrigation, Fit for Life and food combining. I've been to a hypnotist and taken away a tape that I still use to help me sleep. But none of it helped me lose weight.

I went to famous (and not-so-famous) dieticians and nutritionists. I did the Oprah boot camp (which is seriously hardcore), but couldn't stick to it for more than a week. I bought Gillian McKeith. I went up to Carol Vorderman at a do and just said simply, 'Thank you for your detox, Carol, I feel great,' before tucking into pudding. I joined a nutrition home study course and only got to lesson one and couldn't be bothered with the rest of it. I have been a member of a gym on and off for seven years and – although it pains me to say it – if I am really honest I've only been twenty times.

It looks like a hobby, when you see all the diets I've done. I'm a bloody expert. I've spent thousands and thousands of pounds and felt so much heartache and so much pain and so much numbness and so much not really understanding what is going on . . . And I've spent so much time thinking about and trying to work out why, when I am pretty successful in the rest of my life, I couldn't do this one thing. Why wouldn't it happen for me? Couldn't I buy the thing that would make the weight go? Couldn't I wake up and fit into a Jigsaw dress?

I had a happy childhood. I had a bit more flesh on me than most children at school but actually, looking at the pictures now, I was just a happy girl who was an average size. Healthy looking. I didn't think a bit about my size until the 'puppy fat' was noticed by other children (and adults who should have known better). I ate good food. My mum had a thing about tins, and insisted on cooking food from fresh – but we were allowed the occasional treat.

I remember eating pie and chips in front of *Happy Days*.
My sister and I would cut our pies into four. She would eat
her largest bit first. She reckoned she would be full by the time
she got to the smallest bit, and didn't want to leave more than
was strictly necessary. How boring was she? I would leave the
biggest bit until the end. When everyone else was finished, I
would look at my pie with pride. Pie was power. My grandfather
used to say, 'Always leave the table while you've got space for
more,' but I can't remember doing it. Ever.

I remember one particular ballet class. I'd been with the
same school since I was six or seven and I did enjoy it but the
Gaston Payne School of Dance wasn't called the Ghastly Pain
school of dance for nothing. One day when I was ten, I was
busily doing my bit of dancing in a class when Sara, the owner's
daughter, walked up and down the row of us girls by the bar
and said to me in front of everyone, 'Neris Thomas, do you eat
lots of cakes? Because it looks like you do. If you don't stop you
are going to look like the back of a bus.'

I didn't say anything. All I could think was, 'I don't actually
eat many cakes so why is she saying that?', and I kept trying to
work out what she meant by 'the back of a bus'. There were a
few girls sniggering by my side, but I didn't even really register
them at the time. My lovely friend Alison Evans was there to
give me a reassuring little word at the end of the class and make
me feel better. I seemed to attract these kinds of comments
throughout my childhood. I assumed everyone did.

I remember the boys at the back of the bus on the way home
from school who would shout and sing, 'Nelly the Elephant
packed her trunk' whenever I walked on, brilliantly changing
'Nelly' to 'Neris'. I just smiled at them and sat down. It didn't
really bother me that much. I just thought they were a bit mean.
I was happy as I was, and luckily I had my parents at home
telling me to 'rise above it'. But it must have registered. To this
day it's not a song I encourage my daughter to sing.

Puberty changed everything. I became aware of my body in
a new way. I remember seeing a girl called Caroline P.W. in her

swimming costume at the age of eleven, and wondering why I didn't look like that – not an inch of fat on her. I do remember my darling friend at secondary school getting more and more anorexic in front of my eyes and not being able to help her. I didn't understand the fuss back then.

And I remember the school lunches. I just ate the white rolls and butter every day – every single day. Thank goodness I was going home to eat normal food because lunch just consisted of warm white rolls. I still remember them being lovely. I certainly didn't think about nutrition.

I didn't cook myself. I don't think my all-girls' school did domestic science. The school was too busy investing in the new science block.

I avoided PE as much as possible. I remember queuing patiently for the trampoline at an Open Day for the local secondary school. I felt a bit nervous in my tights and leotard, only to step on to the trampoline, and to hear the gym teacher say, 'Now everyone, step back – you might feel the vibrations from this little lady.' What a bastard. But I got through it. It wasn't the worst thing in the world and I was always told how lovely and pretty I was by my mum and dad and sister and I just swallowed the feelings. I was never cross.

By the time school finished, I was still what could be described as an average size: not skinny-mini, but not too big either. It wasn't until university that things changed. In the first year away from home I gained a lot of weight. Not cooking meant my food was a bit limited. I relied on easy things to make. I remember eating a lot of bread. Toast in the morning followed by sandwiches for lunch and pasta for tea. Carbohydrates kept me going for three years. I started to eat chocolate, and the bars just seemed to be getting bigger and bigger. And, of course, so did I.

At university, I had really lovely male friends, who remained just friends. I couldn't quite work out why. I was determined that one day the right boy would like me for who and what I was. I saw no reason to change, and I carried on dreaming that

one day my prince would come. By the end of the first year
at university I was weighing in at fourteen and a half stone.
I glossed over it. Besides, I found girls who obsessed about
food and what they looked like really infuriating and boring.

I wasn't desperate to change but I think I was becoming a bit
more aware of what I looked like. I started eating low-calorie
ready-meals for ease – it seemed like at least I would be sticking
to some kind of regime. I even took myself off to the local
branch of a weight-loss club but found it just too difficult. I do
remember really liking the women in the group, but I was so
disorganized. I was always losing my diet plans and found the
recipes hugely complicated.

I watched Oprah Winfrey every day and got so excited when
I saw her get slim and fit. It just hit a raw nerve. I would cry
during every programme. Something was stirring in me. By the
time I graduated I was still around that fourteen-stone mark.
I went back home just to regroup, but I decided that, finally, at
twenty-one, I wanted to lose the weight. I had been ensconced
in a highly unsuccessful relationship throughout my third year
at university which was so on and off, and I wanted it to be on
so badly that I was on a mission.

For three months I was hardcore. Weight Watchers. Brilliant.
I had three months to go before I would see any of my
university friends. I had a date in September (my close friend's
leaving party as she was off to Australia for a bit) and I knew my
old flame would be there. I wanted to wow him. Back at home,
I was in control. I even started doing exercise classes. I felt safe
– and the weight just dropped off. Even though it was fifteen
years ago, I remember it so clearly – knocking on Jules' front
door, three months on and four stone lighter, and her opening
it and literally not believing what she saw. I was wearing a little
red jacket and jeans. I looked good. 'Wow,' she shrieked, and
all my friends were amazed. The boy I liked couldn't believe it
either . . . but he was later found snogging my friend upstairs.

And at that point I remember consciously deciding to eat
the cake at the party. There was no point in depriving myself.

And there, at that moment, something changed. Despite being thrilled by my transformation, all my hard work went out the window and was quickly overshadowed by my emotions. That pattern of emotional eating has continued on and off, *EastEnders*-style, ever since.

I moved to London and started work in the film industry. It was all so exciting – film sets, late nights and gorgeous actors. But the set catering, lunches out, parties and expense-account dinners weren't ideal for the waistline. The weight crept back on and I didn't get my act together to try to lose it for a few more years when I got fed up with not being able to wear all the clothes I wanted to, and it started to feel uncomfortable. So I dieted.

Again, by being really low calorie I went right down to ten and a half stone (my lowest adult weight). I went on holiday to Bali with my friends and loved it. I felt I had really got it this time. I was in the swing and couldn't believe I would ever go back to my old self. Why would I, when I looked and felt so much better? I was by the pool and looking good. I wasn't even wearing a T-shirt over my swimming costume. Back home, the men seemed to like me more. They started coming out of the woodwork saying, actually, they'd always liked me or that they *would* like me once I lost those pounds . . .

Then, at twenty-eight, I met the man of my dreams, a man that thought then – and still does now – that I'm the most beautiful girl in the world. He really thinks that. By week two I'd practically moved in and we were seriously into our new life together. We were both eating more and more and more. Huge plates of pasta. The three cheese varieties were our favourite. Lots of late night takeaways in front of satellite television. Blissfully in love, the weight came back. But I was okay, now I had found my prince charming.

Over the years I've been with him, Richard has made me feel amazing (sheesh . . . stop the love song on the record player) but once, while I was moaning about my clothes not fitting, he warned me that – at seventeen stone – even though I was the love of his life and he loved me completely – if I put on a lot more weight that he might stop finding me attractive. He still thought I was the most beautiful girl, but he was just being honest. Harsh words that made me so angry I wanted to hit him – I thought he loved me! He still stands by what he said to me that day and says that he is just telling the truth, and saying out loud what every other man thinks. But I thought love was blind. I was confused. And the bastard who is now my husband had hit on a nerve. I was angry.

I wanted to prove everyone wrong – and lose the weight. I started looking for the answer. The secret. And basically I spent the next few years doing just that. I hired Fergie's personal trainer for a day who was great but was way too expensive for me, and I ended up looking a bit of a prat running up and down the staircase in a house with my landlady giggling at the noise from the next room.

I couldn't find a diet that worked for me. Some I only stuck to for a few days, some I stuck to for longer. Sometimes I just bought the book. Then I would feel great relief when the introduction told me that I should read it all the way through before preparing my kitchen and my life for change. Hurrah! But by the time I got to the end of the book I just couldn't be bothered with all the faff.

For my wedding I knew I had a target. I had to do it, so I girded my loins and got down to twelve stone. I got into exercise big time, for the first time ever. I met an amazing woman called Sharon Saker who taught me to love, can you believe it, jogging. I cut out wheat and I really went for it. I had an aim – I had a dress to fit into. I did it, and felt like I glowed for the whole day. I vowed again I wouldn't go back to my old ways.

It lasted until our honeymoon and gradually, you've guessed it, the weight came back.

For the last few years I've spent my time procrastinating, trying to muster up the energy to change. 'If I lose two pounds a week – no, maybe I could push it to three pounds a week – every week for the next six weeks then by the time it's so and so's wedding I'll look okay.' I kept on smiling and procrastinating, and after a year of thinking I'd postpone getting pregnant until I had lost all my weight I gave up on the notion and got pregnant straight away.

We had our beautiful precious daughter. But our lives were then taken over by her being extremely ill. We spent a month living in Intensive Care and all I can remember was going to the vending machine and eating chocolate. My husband later told me he was going to the vending machine on the floor below. Eating was my only comfort.

Things thankfully, and incredibly, eventually got better, but when, weeks later, we emerged from the hospital, I weighed myself and I was topping the scales at just under eighteen stone.

I ate and ate, but we were home and that was all that mattered. I tried to carry on, but I think I had just lost my oomph. I'd felt frustrated and sad before, but I had never lost my spirit. By the time I had a one-year-old baby, my husband had an exciting new job. Having always been a very sociable person, I found myself making excuses to get out of meeting his new colleagues – for example, saying to him that his Christmas party clashed with my friends coming around – because my overwhelming feeling was that I was actually a bit embarrassing for him.

I wanted people to see him and think he was great and if they saw me they would think less of him. I thought that I would let him down. I had been overweight off and on and off and on for sixteen years but I think losing my oomph was the thing that made me really think. That hadn't happened before. I felt that I really had to do something about this and suddenly the years felt like they had passed really quickly and all the people I read about in *Slimming World* and the other weight-loss magazines seemed to be twenty-one when they reached their goal and I felt really jealous of them.

My force of nature, my all-or-nothing character, got me into this mess and it also kept me in it, because I wouldn't be told what I should be or what I should do. It has taken nearly twenty years to work out what I was doing wrong, and where I was going wrong. Finally the time had arrived to sort it out for once and for all. Who would have thought that India and me sitting in a café, chatting about everything, and then talking about how we both really had to do something about our weight would lead to me changing for ever. Never to go back. I promise.

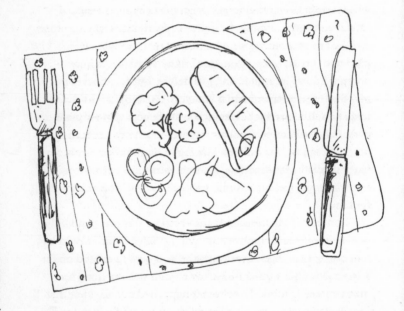

2. Lessons We Have Learned

The million-dollar question is: what happened this time around that hadn't happened in the past (for Neris), or that suddenly spurred me (India) into action after so many years? I'd been overweight for well over a decade, and Neris, as we have just seen, had really struggled, on and off, for much longer. At this late stage, it might have been easier to give up, go with the flow, and live in tent dresses, finally reconciled to a life of lardiness. And yet here we are. How? What happened?

Well, we had each other. This is not to be underestimated: it was absolutely central to our weight loss, both in terms of kick-starting it and when it came to carrying on – and to getting back in the zone when one or the other of us had wandered off (because yes, we fully expect you to be human and go off-piste every now and then. We'll get to that later). The reason why diet programmes such as Weight Watchers work so well for some people is partly the strong social element. Nobody wants to feel lonely. Fat and lonely is even worse: the combination of being fat and feeling isolated in, and by, your fatness is simply fatal and resolution-sapping. There is something enormously comforting in knowing you're with people in the same boat, who have been where you've been, who know what you're talking about, who know what it's like.

We strongly recommend finding yourself a diet buddy. Be sensible: try not to pick your most competitive friend. A mild degree of competition is no bad thing, but you don't want a control-freak as a buddy, or someone who cheats like mad and starves themselves, or starts spending six hours a day in the gym so they lose faster than you. If there's no suitable candidate around, and even if there is, think of this book as that buddy. Seriously. Imagine it's a person. Ask it questions: use the Index. Really get to know it. This book doesn't just tell you what to do: it holds your hand at every stage of the way, gives you a nice hug when you've done well, and gives you an extra-big one when you're struggling.

(Maybe you want to know how Neris and I first met. We were always at the same parties wearing identical clothes. We were both expert at shopping for our size, but because the choice is so limited, we kept bumping into each other identically dressed, like Tweedledum and Tweedledee. We were quite well dressed, I have to say – because between us we had decades of experience and expertise. (There are tips on clothes, and on making the most of what you've got, whatever size you are now, on pages 102–4.)

Neris and I had both come to the stage where enough was enough. It is always being said of addicts of all kinds that they need to hit rock bottom before they can build themselves up again, and the same applied to us. I don't want to sound melodramatic, or to make light of people's addictions to narcotics or alcohol, but we were, after all, addicted to quantities of food, and in particular to carbohydrates. And we did hit rock bottom: me in Selfridges, Neris in the comfort of her own home. We had a moment of revelation, and the revelation was this: the thing about weight is that it doesn't have to be the boss of you. Even if it's been your boss for years, or decades. Even if you're in total despair because you have more than five stone to lose. Even if you think, ah, sod it, what's the point.

Have you had enough? You wouldn't have picked up this book if you hadn't.

▸ Do you want to feel fantastic, every day?
▸ Do you want to wear clothing of the kind you can't imagine owning, let alone fitting into, in a million years – and look great in it? Because you can, you know. It is a goal that is entirely possible to attain.
▸ Do you want to regain control over the one aspect of your life you think you have no control over?

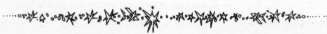

Of course you do. Yes, yes, yes and yes, you're saying, like Meg Ryan in *When Harry Met Sally*.

Well, good. Because that's exactly what we're going to help you to do. And it's going to work for you, just like it worked for us.

Now, on to the trickier stuff. We came to understand why we ate, or overate, and before we get going properly you need to understand why you do it, too. It has absolutely nothing to do with hunger, needless to say. Your brain may interpret that empty, dissatisfied feeling as hunger pangs, but that's not what they are. And you're not going to get anywhere, frankly, until you've identified exactly why you overeat.

Why We Eat Too Much

Because we're unhappy. We can be massively depressed, or microscopically annoyed by something completely trivial, but if we associate food with comfort, we'll eat. We both ate if our children were unwell, and we both ate if the plumber had failed to turn up. We ate because it was raining. We ate because we'd had a titchy argument with our partners. We ate because we'd stubbed our toe, or because somebody was sick in hospital. The gravity or otherwise of the situation had nothing to do with it. We ate because, for whatever reason, we felt sad.

Because we're happy. For example, I (India) have always associated food with celebration. It's partly a cultural thing – I'm half Indian, and all the women in my family express their love through cooking, and through feeding you ('Eat, eat, I made it especially for you'). I don't know if white Anglo-Saxon Protestants do this too, but Jews certainly do, and Muslims, and the French, and the Italians, and pretty much everyone else I can think of. Food is a celebration of life and as such is central to certain cultures – not because they need to eat to live, but because food becomes a metaphor for everything good and loving and enjoyable about life. This is a lovely thing; I'm not knocking it. But it does create powerful associations that aren't especially helpful if you develop a problem with your weight. You start to believe that ALL food is about love. It isn't. Does food reinforce happiness? No.

Because it's a habit. Like smoking, or twirling your hair. Eating becomes a knee-jerk response. Got a spare ten minutes? Have a wee snack with your cup of tea. Watching telly? Have a biscuit. Out shopping? Don't forget to stop for coffee and sandwiches.

Because we're bored. Fatal, this one. Calamitous. Especially if you're at home all day, endlessly peering into the fridge or making toast to accompany your cup of tea. Some of us can't even read a magazine without having something to snack on. I've had many a bath with a bar of chocolate alongside me. When my children were small and I was up half the night, I'd sometimes eat in between their night feeds. And so it goes on.

Because we're already fat. The thin person's mindset says: 'Eat something else? Why would I want to do that? I just had dinner.' The fat person's mindset says, 'Okay. So, rationally, I know I'm not hungry. I ate a big dinner two hours ago. But I'm sitting here not quite knowing what to do with myself, so I might as well nip down to the kitchen and find something to pick at. I know it's not a good idea, because I don't need the calories and I'll get fat. But I'm already fat. So it's not going to make a huge amount of difference.' I thought this for years on end. My thought process went: 'Bloody hell, I've put on so much weight. It's really grim. I must do something about it. But not now, obviously, because who on earth starts a diet at eleven o'clock at night? No, I'll begin tomorrow. So I might as well have a cheese toastie.' Did the cheese toastie make me feel better? What do you think?

Because we have a weird empty feeling. We don't like the feeling, and what you do with an empty thing is fill it up. Here's a thing: the weird empty feeling has absolutely nothing to do

CHAPTER TWO   40   LESSONS WE HAVE LEARNED

with food. NOT A THING. It has to do with dissatisfaction or unhappiness or stress or worry, and possibly feelings of all four because of your appearance. But it does not have to do with appetite.

Because we believe the crap we're told. And why shouldn't we, when advertising is so sophisticated and psychologically astute? We believe that chocolate bars are a wonderful way to reward yourself. We believe life wouldn't be complete without balls of dough fried in oil and sprinkled with white sugar. We're told these foods are 'naughty' or 'sinful', and naturally that makes them even more attractive and desirable. You know how we laugh at how little children are mesmerized by TV ads for this or that must-have (supposedly) toy? We shouldn't laugh. We're exactly the same. We watch a lovingly, almost pornographically photographed shot of a milkshake (made with pig fat and sugar) and feel compelled to get in our car and drive to the nearest fast-food outlet.

Because we're greedy. And we've probably messed our bodies around so much that they're as confused as we are about what does and doesn't constitute feeling full. It's important to address greediness, and we will. Because the truth is, we're not 'big-boned' or 'well-built'. We weren't obese babies. We don't suffer from some bizarre biological malfunction that causes us to get fatter and fatter for no reason. Get it into your head: we're not *supposed* to look this way. We got fat. The totally brilliant thing is, we can get un-fat.

You may, of course, have some reasons of your own to add to the ones above, but they're broadly accurate, we think, for the majority of people. Now, don't just turn the page. Re-read the above. Nodding in agreement is one thing, but you need to go further: you need to really understand (sorry if we're sounding bossy. Bear with us. This is important).

Get this into your head.

If you're feeling sad, eating does not make you happy.
Eating does not make the bad thing go away. Sure, you feel
better for five or ten minutes. And then you feel much worse.
You're still sad about whatever you were sad about, and now
you're sad about having stuffed your face as well. This is not
a result.

**If you're feeling happy, eating does not make you
happier.** Would you have enjoyed your wedding day more
if you'd been snacking on doughnuts as you walked down the
aisle? Do the mothers of new-born babies feel compelled to
eat pies as they gaze into their newborns' eyes? Would hot
sex be hotter if you had a tub of Pringles to hand? Please.

Eating is not a habit. Nothing you do to yourself is ever
a habit. You *always* have a choice.

Eating does not alleviate boredom. We think it often
causes it, because eating the wrong thing can make you feel
incredibly tired and listless.

You don't need us to point out that eating because you're
already fat – the 'oh, sod it' factor – is not going to make you
thinner. Eating because you can't be bothered to do anything
about your weight is something we both understand really well.
It is born of despair. And there's no need to despair, because
even if you're really seriously overweight, you can lose that
weight. You can. We know. We did it.

The weird empty feeling isn't about hunger. It is about
feeling dissatisfied, whether it's because you're having a bad
hair day or because you've just realized your marriage sucks.
Addressing the issue will lead to a resolution. Eating won't.
Really examine those ads. Think about that cultural
conditioning. The woman whose sugar-laden yogurt is so good
that she forgets to have sex with the dishy man waiting for her?
Yeah, right. Somebody's having a laugh, no? At your expense.
Get wise to it.

Yes, we are greedy. Accept it. You're not going to starve on
this diet. You can still be greedy. But in a good way, not an
incontinent, out-of-control fat person's way.

Chances are that if you've ever forgotten to eat – and no, it's not something we've made a habit of, either – it was because you were too busy having a good time. Too busy full stop doesn't count, otherwise there would be no overweight office workers or stay-at-home mothers. You need to be busy *and* loving whatever it is you're doing to forget about food: for example, nobody has fantastic sex and pauses in the middle to reflect on how they're really starving, actually. You don't take to the floor on your wedding day thinking, 'I could murder a Cornish pasty.' You don't watch your child being Star Number Two in the school Christmas play and find your mind wandering to the question of jumbo bags of Twiglets. Or maybe you do – it's all subjective. Our point is that when you are fully, 100 per cent engaged with doing something you enjoy, whatever it is, appetite takes a back seat.

Even if this doesn't happen very often, chances are that it has at least happened occasionally. Focus on that time. What it tells you is this: the food you eat to excess is a crutch, and that crutch is not always necessary, since you don't need it when you're really enjoying yourself.

Here's a thought: you think you're eating to relieve your boredom, to ease your anxiety, to soothe your fevered brow, to calm yourself down or to rev yourself up. You're not. You are eating to punish yourself.

This is a bit of a head-fuck. You think you're being nice to yourself when you overeat. But you aren't. You're making yourself fat and unhealthy, and in the process you're making yourself feel terrible as soon as you've finished eating that pot of ice cream or that fried cheese sandwich. You are being horrible to yourself, is the truth of the matter. And the really mad thing about it is, you are punishing yourself for having no control over events (the thing, whatever it was, that drove you to the kitchen in the first place) by losing control of yourself. Do you see? It's a crazy lack-of-control double whammy.

Here's an example: it's after breakfast, which you've had, and you're feeling mighty pissed off. The children's rooms are like

're old enough to tidy after themselves. Then
the dog and bang your shin. The phone rings: it's
share the school run with, telling you that she's
can't, in fact, collect the kids from school today
has a sudden and unscheduled work appointment.
now feeling intensely irritated with the shape your day
is taking, and it's only 10am. It starts raining, and you have to
walk the dog. Lead in hand, you autopilot down to the kitchen,
flick the kettle on and make a cup of tea. There's an open packet
of the children's Jaffa Cakes calling your name from the shelf.
You sit down and eat every single one. Better now?

No. Of course not. On top of your shin and the bedrooms and
the stupid dog and the inept friend and having to go out in a
Noah-worthy downpour, you've just eaten a gigantic amount
of biscuits. How does that help? How is that being nice to
yourself? What you've done is added to the general crapness of
the day, because now on top of everything else you feel like a fat
pig. Great. Fan-fucking-tastic.

It is really essential to grasp this point. You comfort eat. You
think comfort eating is a way of showing yourself some love.
It's not. It's the exact opposite. And just because you love food
doesn't mean it loves you back. It's not saying, 'Ahh, kissy-kissy,
I love you so much.' It's saying, 'Christ, there she goes again,
shovelling me down. All right, Tubs? Shall we have seconds?
Yeah, thought so. Any day now she's going to break this chair
with the weight of her arse.'

No matter how much spin you put on it, no matter how
hilarious you are when you talk about yourself and food, no
matter how brilliant you've become at the self-deprecating
jokes, the truth is that overeating is a form of self-dislike, or, to
put it less brutally, self-unease. You know the L'Oréal ad? You're
the opposite. You don't really believe you're worth it. Even if
– *especially* if – to everyone else, you're the acme of confidence
and strength.

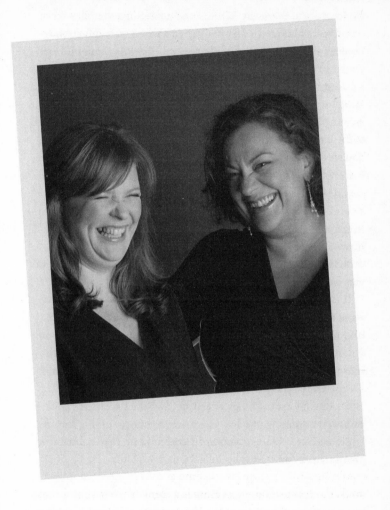

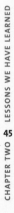

Here Are Some Good Ways of Showing Yourself Real Love

Go for a walk. Seriously. Whenever people suggested this to us, either in real life or in diet books, we wanted to laugh at how lame and prissy it sounded. What kind of a pussy suggestion is walking? This is what we thought of going for walks: marginally preferable to touching a poo with bare hands, but only just. Walk vs. Jaffa Cake: no contest, right? But bear with us. Give it a try. We're not talking a five-mile hike here: we're talking a quick walk to the shops, or to the park, if there's one nearby, or even a brisk trot around the block. Quite apart from its many health benefits, which we'll get to later, walking clears your head in a manner that sometimes seems miraculous. Nothing is as bad after a walk as it seemed before it (they're particularly brilliant in the middle of arguments). Obviously, there's a leap of faith involved here, but you'll have to trust us. Your head will feel a million times clearer, and your problems, whatever they were, will feel smaller or even, with luck, insignificant.

Have a cat-nap. Nothing is so important that it can't wait ten minutes. Lying down and closing your eyes not only energizes you but also has the most marvellously soothing effect on the mind. Take deep breaths. You'll feel better. Have a bath. Baths are bliss, especially if you're more used to having a shower. Buy some delicious things to put in the bath – scented oils or bubbles. Loofah your back. Lie there, soaking, sniffing the air appreciatively. Relax. If you have longer, read a book until you go all wrinkly and pruny.

Find your favourite song and dance around like a loony for three and a half minutes. Yes, it's an old women's magazine favourite. But it's also a guaranteed energizer, plus you feel all giggly for looking like a prat, and the giggliness lasts for some time. If you feel self-conscious, draw the curtains and do it in the dark.

Phone a friend – preferably the diet buddy we mentioned earlier. Have a gossip. Tell some jokes. Arrange to meet up later in the week.

Get as extravagant as your time or purse situation allows. Go shopping. Take yourself for coffee, and don't spoil the occasion by wolfing down a couple of cakes. You're taking care of yourself, not giving a spoiled toddler a treat. Sitting down with a cup of tea and the new issue of your favourite magazine is a lovely thing to do. Have a manicure. Get your hair blow-dried, or blow-dry it yourself (this makes us feel incredibly happy, for some reason – far happier than twenty minutes with a big brush and a hairdryer ought to warrant).

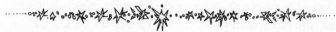

Watch an Inspiring Film
▶ *Rocky* – because it's brilliant . . . but only the first one
▶ *Forrest Gump* – just to get you walking and running
▶ *When Harry Met Sally* – just to be like Meg Ryan was then
▶ *Billy Elliot* – we really do want to boogie
▶ *Strictly Ballroom* – you'll never be able to sit still again through 'Love Is In The Air'

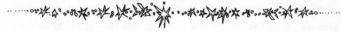

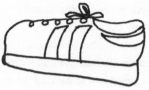

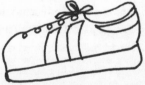

Notice we're not suggesting re-decorating the children's rooms, or baking them a cake for a treat, or doing the ironing. All of these activities, and others like them, aren't about you. The point of this exercise is to be nice to yourself. It is exclusively about you. It doesn't mean you're a slattern, or a selfish monster who doesn't love her family. It means you're learning to value yourself as highly as you value your loved ones. And there's nothing wrong with that – quite the opposite. If you'd like to read more about how, sometimes, selfishness is quite nice, turn to page 57.

While we're on the subject of love, here's a little more on one of the things we briefly touched on earlier, namely families that communicate through food. You'll either immediately know what we're talking about, or you won't have a clue, in which case you can probably skip this bit. Though we wouldn't, if we were you. The penny might drop.

Does this scenario sound at all familiar? You're overweight. You've been noticeably overweight for a while. You go and visit your mum.[2] She knew you were coming, so she's been cooking. She's pulled out all the stops. She's made you a feast. Isn't that nice? 'Eat, eat,' she says. 'I've been cooking all day/night.'

Aah, you think to yourself. That's so lovely! And you sit down, and you start eating. Your mother encourages you to have seconds. Thirds, even – 'Oh, just this tiny little slice won't hurt, I made it especially for you.' So you do. Nothing like your mum's cooking, is there?

Or it can go like this: she's made you the aforementioned feast. It's *quite* nice. Nice of her to spend the time and effort, but kind of odd to have baked three kinds of cheesecake, or samosas, or whatever, when you've explicitly told her you were trying to lose weight. And now she's urging you to eat it, and her face is going all sad and crumpled when you're saying you'll only have a small piece. Oh God, now you feel bad. You feel

[2] We're not picking on mums, though they're more likely to do this than your dad. But insert whatever you need to here – mother, father, brother, sister, auntie, uncle, granny, grandpa or, more often than not, friend (so-called).

guilty. Whatever, you think. I'll eat the damnthing
tomorrow. As you swallow the first delicious mouthf...
yourself, 'Is my mum deaf, or something? Because she
I'm watching my weight. Weird. Ah well.'

Or like this: same situation. The difference this time is th.
your mum absolutely knows you're overweight, and is always
urging you to do something about it, much to your irritation.
You go and visit. She's made a feast. The feast is lavish in your
eyes – whether it's a three-course banquet or a jumbo portion
of cod and chips – and one glance tells you it's super-fattening.
You raise your eyebrows. 'Oh, I know,' she smiles. 'But once in
a while won't hurt.' And you wonder to yourself why she has
knowingly cooked you the food you both know you shouldn't
be eating. 'Wow,' you think to yourself. 'There's something not
quite right here.'

That third scenario is the worst, but actually none of them
are great if you have a weight problem. As we were saying
above, there are entire cultures – entire countries, in fact
entire continents – that habitually behave in this way. It's not
always a bad thing, though I have come to the conclusion that
demonstrating one's love through food is only valid if it is
demonstrated in other ways also. Put brutally, it's easy to cook
(or to nip to the baker's to buy a cream cake). Pretty much
anyone can do it. What's less easy is to say – for example – 'I'm
still feeling quite cross with you over such-and-such, but I love
you, whatever you do.' Food can be about love, of course, and in
normal situations it usually is. But it can also be about avoiding
the real issue – about replacing emotional sustenance with
physical sustenance, i.e. food. And that, my dears, is often how
and where emotional eating begins. And it can last a lifetime.

Let me explain. Say I was cross with my (not-fat) teenage
son for having a messy room and coming home late on a school
night. I could do two things. I could sit him down, explain that I
was really pretty furious, listen to his side of the story, persuade
him to listen to mine, and try to reach a happy resolution so we
could both sleep easily in our beds that night. Or I could think,

I can't be bothered with this again. I'll just sulk for a bit, so he knows I'm cross with him.' By lunchtime the next day, I'd feel guilty and there would be a horrible atmosphere in the house. So I'd make him his favourite pudding, or pancakes for brunch, by way of an olive branch.

In families that don't have food issues, that might work perfectly well. In families that do, it would be a disaster, especially if I'd started this technique when my child was only a few years old, and especially if my child were overweight. We all do it, up to a point, with the doling out of sweeties or other sugar-laden 'treats', when we're feeling we haven't been as nice to our children as we might have been. But some families take it much further, and if you can't deal with it, then it's catastrophic.

What can you do about it? Well, that depends. We're not going to suggest you take your whole family and/or friends off for a spot of group therapy, because as suggestions go, that one's a bit too hardcore for most of us. No, all you really need to do is be aware of the situation. Knowledge is power. If you are able to calmly identify what's going on, and to think to yourself, 'I see. This is what's happening. It's part of a pattern that's been going on for years, and it is no longer a pattern I want to involve myself in,' then you're halfway there (give yourself a massive pat on the back, please). Be calm. Don't start frothing at the mouth and giving your loved ones a lecture about emotional eating. It's all about you, remember?

Don't give the people who encourage you to comfort eat any ammunition. If you feel that you're surrounded by them, ignore our admonition to do this diet in secret, and tell everyone you're on a diet, tell them what you can and can't eat, and explain that, come hell or high water, you will not go off-course, even for one meal. Don't apologize for yourself by prefixing any of this with 'I know it's a bore, but . . . ' What are you apologizing for? Getting in shape? Being good to yourself? The person you're talking to will probably say that they'll make something especially for you, something you can eat. Politely thank them, and explain that this won't be necessary. YOU are in control of what you put in your mouth. Nobody else.

You don't need special food, as you'll see when we get to the nuts and bolts of this diet. Unless you have friends or family who exist solely on carbohydrates, there will always be something you can eat. You don't need other people to create special menus for you – you're not an invalid. You don't even need to draw attention to your way of eating. If the worst comes to the worst, you'll go home feeling slightly peckish. So what, really? At home you'll have a fridge stocked with delicious food you can eat. Besides, we can all act, up to a point. Whatever you do, don't look miserable, even if you feel it at first (you won't feel it for long, we promise. Taking control is incredibly empowering, to use a horrible word). Eat what you can eat, cheerfully. Compliment the cook. For God's sake don't whinge about how you wish you could have the chips. Whinging, or looking glum, reinforces the negative and self-sabotaging message that you are somehow punishing yourself. Which is mad, because you are doing the exact opposite. You are celebrating how fantastic you're going to look and feel. Whinging also gives your host ammunition – they'll think, 'She'll never stick it out. I'm going to ignore everything she's saying.' Being confident and cheerful has the opposite effect. It makes your host think, 'Oh. She's serious.'

By doing this – explaining what the diet involves, and eating only what you are allowing yourself to eat – you are putting out the powerful message that from today onwards, when it comes to food, you are the boss. You are in control. You're no longer going to eat food that makes you fat out of politeness, or out of weariness, or because you want to show X or Y that you love them by eating their food. Take them a bunch of flowers instead. It's much easier on the waistline. Do you now understand how and why you overeat? It's okay if you don't, but if that's the case, please re-read this chapter. Understanding patterns of behaviour is essential if we are going to break them. If you're confident that you've got the basic idea, and if you recognize your overeating triggers, you're ready to turn the page. That means you're ready to embark on our diet. And *that* means you're about to take the first step to becoming thin/slim/healthy.

You'll see a real difference in two weeks. Keep hold of that thought.

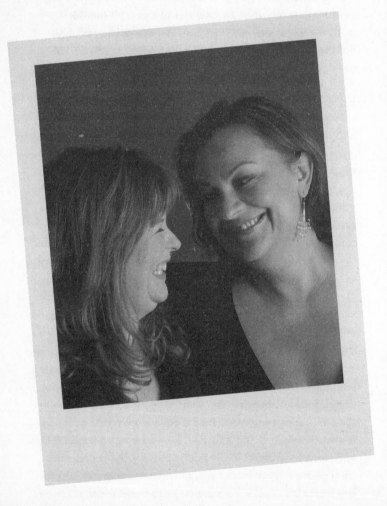

3. Before You Set Off

It is an unfortunate fact of life that when you are trying to diet, obstacles sprout up like mushrooms – and we don't just mean your children's half-empty packet of Wotsits lying temptingly on the kitchen table (though there's always that, too). We think it's a good idea to identify possible pitfalls in advance of them occurring, and to develop some strategies to deal with them.

If you are worried about a specific upcoming event, turn to page 61 for a detailed index of how to cope in many given situations, such as parties, the pub, or Christmas dinner. What we have found far more troubling – and troublesome – than the odd stray sweetie, or the sudden overwhelming urge to think, 'Ah, bugger it, I'll just eat this sticky toffee pudding, and start again tomorrow,' are other people. As the writer and critic Mary McCarthy once said of someone who made a habit of always helpfully pointing out her bad reviews to her, 'There's always friends.'

Girlfriends, in particular, can be very peculiar about your dieting. They're pleased for you – up to a point. We've lost track of the number of times we've both been told, by well-meaning 'friends', that we didn't need to lose another pound and were utterly gorgeous just as we were (at fourteen and a half stone). Now, either these friends are so blinded with love that they can't see you as you really are, or, we're sorry to say, the idea of you controlling your biggest vice – your overeating – makes them distinctly uncomfortable.

Women are strange creatures. When I (India) got divorced, many of my girlfriends suddenly got very possessive of their husbands. I can honestly say that, to me, the majority of these husbands were monstrous gargoyles (I'm sure they spoke very highly of me, too). I wouldn't have touched them with a very long stick. They were my nice girlfriends' inexplicably dull, unattractive, or both, spouses, and over the years I'd learned to put up with them, and they with me. And yet, suddenly, their wives were behaving as though their fat, bald, braying, comainducingly boring husbands were Brad Pitt, and I was some sex-crazed, frenziedly lustful femme fatale, instead of a knackered single mother who'd really rather be asleep, but who'd come round for a drink because it seemed rude to say 'no' three times in a row. Weird, or what? But it happened with alarming frequency.

It's the same thing with weight. People don't like too much movement around the status quo. You're supposed to be fat, they think – it's just how you are. If you wanted to do something about it, surely you would have done it by now. No, you must be really comfortable in your skin, and happy with your lot. So you get pigeonholed: you sit in your little box, which says 'My fat friend', and you're not really allowed to jump out. People are threatened by change, and they are especially threatened by change in their close friends. This is particularly true of people who aren't especially happy, and for whom the smallest change can tip the balance in a negative way. For these people, the fact that you have done something and confronted an issue – your weight – head-on can seem threatening. But, do you know, that's their business. It's not yours.

So it shouldn't surprise you that the friend who's offered to cook you dinner 'forgets' about your eating plan, and puts a chocolate cake in front of you for pudding. You shouldn't be too shocked when, out for the evening, your friend urges you to eat something you're not supposed to, 'just this once'. And neither should you be surprised if the same friend – or another: this has happened to both of us with a variety of people – suddenly tells you that you're getting too thin, when you both know perfectly well that you've got another couple of stones to go before you're anywhere near a healthy weight for your height. It's not just your skinny friends: your overweight friends are more than likely to be incredibly dismissive of your dieting plans, because of course the act of you dieting reminds them that they could do with losing weight too; that you're doing something about your problem and they're not. We know this to be true because we've done it ourselves. As for colleagues: no one should have to put up with the nosy woman who sits opposite you and makes a point of investigating, and commenting on, your packed lunch every day.

This sabotaging *will* happen in one way or another, no matter how charming, lovely and supportive your friends are. And we suggest quite a radical solution to it. This is not to tell anyone that you're on a diet – excepting, of course, your designated diet buddy, if you have one.

Dieting is like giving up smoking: if you involve other people and make a great big song and dance about it, anything they say – from 'How boring of you' to 'Congratulations' – is potentially irritating and anxiety-causing. This is because you now feel that you're not just dieting for yourself, but for other people, and naturally their input matters to you. And by telling them about it, you're giving them licence to comment.

Do you really want their comments? Think about it. Probably not. If the person who originally said, 'Congratulations,' now says, 'Oh, go on, this little piece of bread won't hurt you,' a weird thing happens psychologically. You think, 'This person is on my side. And yet they're telling me to have the bread. That means it must be okay.' Conversely, the person who says, 'How boring,' is not on your side from the off, and is unlikely to be helpful. Why not simply avoid both scenarios by keeping quiet about the whole project? Life's too short.

You need to remember that you are doing this diet for you. You're in charge of yourself – nobody else is. Only you can influence what you eat – nobody else can. Losing weight is your responsibility, and no one else's. So we suggest you quietly get on with it. That way, nobody will be expecting you to succeed, and nobody will be expecting you to fail, which removes an enormous amount of stress and pressure. Nobody will stare at your plate and say, 'Doesn't look much like diet food to me.' Nobody will say, 'Should you really be eating that?' or 'But it's low fat, you can have it,' or 'I don't believe in diets. You should just exercise more,' or any of the other little things that can drive you up the wall. And nobody will cause you to feel humiliated in public by loudly announcing, 'She's on a diet' (cue everyone turning round to stare at Miss Tubs).

So our advice, which you are free to ignore, is to keep schtum. Aside from anything else, it will stop you from turning into the incredibly tiresome kind of woman who's always thinking and talking about food. You might even want to keep it from your partner. Does he really need to know? Wouldn't it drive you crazy if he started commenting all the time about what you're eating, and looked all disappointed if you slipped up? (This last scenario is so demoralizing and stressful that it might very well make you give up altogether.) The same thing applies with your children: do their mates, coming round to tea, really need to know that you're on a diet? You might as well wear a sticker on your head saying, 'Hi! I'm a Fat Mum.' We say no. And given that you can eat or prepare the food your family normally eats, doing the diet quietly and noiselessly is entirely feasible. You all have the roast pork, but only they have the mash. You have some cheese instead of pudding. Unless your family are directly related to Hercule Poirot, they probably won't even notice.

If it becomes impossible to keep quiet about the diet, i.e. if someone asks you about it directly, say something vague like, 'I thought I'd try and eat more healthily for a couple of days.' Remember: you're doing this for yourself. And, you know, you don't need help from anybody, apart from your trusted diet buddy, or this book.

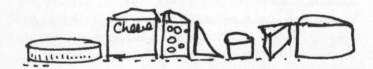

4. How to Be More Selfish

Oprah Winfrey, who knows a thing or two about losing weight, says that you can only begin to do so once you are completely at ease and comfortable with yourself. In hideous Californian self-help speak, that means you need to love yourself before you can change yourself. And while we may gag a little bit at the way that last sentence is phrased, we have to admit that what the hallowed Ms Winfrey says is true. If you start off from a place of self-loathing – as so many diet books encourage women to do, to say nothing of the media in general – then we believe your chances of failure automatically sky-rocket.

We didn't think we were monstrous blimps when we decided to embark on this eating plan. Well, we may have thought it for a moment or two, but we didn't believe in our hearts that being overweight meant that we were useless human beings. Not for a moment – not even for a nanosecond. We believed, or came to believe, that we were doing ourselves a serious disservice by not addressing our fat problem, which is a different thing altogether, and a more rational one. We liked ourselves enough to do something about it, and we want you to like yourself too. You're going to like yourself a whole lot more when you're the weight you want to be, true. But you need to start off from a good place if you're going to succeed with our way of eating.

Here is a box. Fill it with things you like about yourself – you need to include a minimum of ten. Nobody else is ever going to see it, so don't be shy. If you think you're funny, or clever, or cute, write it down. If you know you're a great cook, or a great mother, or a kind friend, stick it in the box. If you're generous, or green-fingered, or patient, or gentle, or good with cats, get it down. It doesn't matter whether the qualities you like in yourself are big or small – just grab a pen and fill in the box.

Actually, I'm Pretty Great. Here Are Some Reasons Why:

1 _____
2 _____
3 _____
4 _____
5 _____
6 _____
7 _____
8 _____
9 _____
10 _____

See? You *are* great. And the wonderful thing is that within a relatively short amount of time, you're going to look as good as you are possibly capable of looking. We want you to enter this next, new phase of your life feeling gung-ho about the possibilities, not feeling, 'Oh, whatever, I'll give it a go.' Please, please believe us when we say that if we could do this, so can you. We were lazy, tired, busy, really not into dieting, and we lost five stone each. And truly, if we could do it, so could anyone. Including you.

Peaceful and confident is the frame of mind you're aiming for. Stop criticizing yourself for having become fat, for having no willpower, or whatever. Pat yourself on the back instead for having picked up this book.

Congratulate yourself for embarking on this project. Tell yourself the truth, which is that there is no reason why you should fail. You will only fail if you expect to fail – if you think, 'Oh, I'm crap at diets, it'll never work.' That is what we used to think, ten stone ago. If you expect to succeed, there is absolutely nothing that stands in your way. Your only obstacle is your own negative thinking. When you see foods you aren't yet allowed, don't mope and think, 'I wish I could have that, but I can't. Therefore I am being deprived.' Try and replace the thought with, 'By not having that, I am giving myself a huge present – major weight loss.' Here's a naff American motivational saying for you: nothing tastes as good as thin feels. Naff, but true. There is simply no way that the pleasure you might get from eating a doughnut could even begin to compare to the pleasure you feel when you've dropped four dress sizes, or when you realize, as I (India) did, that I am thinner at forty than I was at twenty-five. Nothing I could eat could have the same effect on my spirits. The end result is *so* worth the little (and they are little) sacrifices you have to make along the way.

Neris had spent most of her adult life trying to get this right and it was only when she realized it was her choice to be unhappy and fat, or happy and thinner, that it all clicked into place. **And at the end of the day, none of this is really about food. It's about the way you choose to live your life – unhappy and fat, or happier and thinner.** It's a no-brainer. Once your head – or heart – is fully engaged, you can make things easier for yourself by becoming happier with the way you look. That's the way you look right now, today. Accept it, before you kiss it goodbye. You may not love your body, but it's looked after you. It's kept you healthy. It's maybe borne some children. It's your friend, not your enemy. So at this early stage, before you do anything else, we'd like you to reward it.

Try not to skulk around in fat people's clothes any more. There's a whole lot more coming up about dressing for your size, but for now, stop wearing the clothes that hide you the most. They may hide your flab, but chances are they also hide what you are really about – your spirit, your life force, your *joie de vivre*. Be proud of yourself. You're about to do an amazing thing. Look like you mean business!

Nobody's ever too fat for really good makeup – and my goodness, it really makes a difference. Have a look at your makeup bag. Chuck anything that you've not used for six months or so. Pare everything down to the bare minimum, and practise with what you're left with. Give yourself a makeover. It's not hard, it costs nothing, and if you don't like it, you can

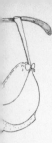

wash it off. It sounds too feeble to be true, but something as simple as wearing new eye makeup – or old eye makeup applied in a new way – can boost your confidence to an enormous extent. Give yourself a new look.

We also recommend that you buy yourself some decent underwear before you even begin the diet. The vast majority of women in Britain wear the wrong bra size, and if you're overweight, wearing the right size can make the most amazing difference to your upper half. With the wrong bra, it's easy to have a bosom that appears to meld seamlessly into your stomach, thus giving you a ridiculous, spherical torso, with no waist and no shape. A properly-fitted bra can solve this problem in one fell swoop – always a majorly cheering development. The same applies to knickers. If you carry fat around your middle, please invest in some control pants. Marks & Spencer's Magic Knickers (www.marksandspencer.com) come highly recommended, but there are a wide variety of other models available in your local department store; we also like the vast array of control garments made by the US brand Spanx (available online from www.mytights.com or www.figleaves. com). These really work. In extreme cases, it is possible for a woman to drop a dress size by wearing the right, well-fitting foundation garments.

In other diet books you would have been in the food section by page ten, but the reason this diet worked for us is that it's necessary to address all of these other issues we've been talking about . . . this is not just a food plan. If it was just about what went into your mouth then it would be easy. Everyone would be slim.

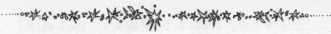

We're almost ready to go. Before we kick off, here is an emergency guide. If you find yourself facing one of the following events at any stage during the diet, just turn to the designated page for help and advice on exactly what to do.

Going to a party **pages 195–197**
Eating in the office **page 93**
Going to the pub **page 198**
Going to a wedding **page 196**
Going to a funeral **page 197**
Eating out in restaurants **page 105 and 198**
Eating in (takeaways) **page 144**
Eating abroad **page 198**
Packed lunches **page 93**
Eating at friends' **page 197**
Children's parties **page 196**
Christmas **page 199**
Preparing a dinner party **page 185–7**
Girls' night out **page 218–9**
Falling off the wagon **pages 163–67, 216–219**

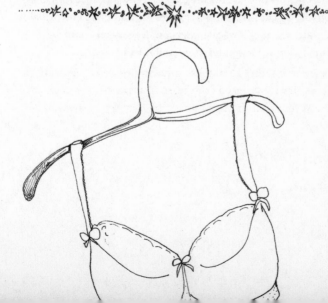

5. Neris and India's Idiot-Proof Diet

Put at its most basic, this is a high-protein, low-carb diet. Eating more protein and fewer carbs than we're used to results in the body using its own stores of fat for fuel. That means you're burning your own fat twenty-four hours a day, seven days a week. And *that* means you're doing some serious shrinking.

We said low-carb, not no-carb. You will be eating carbs, only they'll be good ones, which means GI-friendly ones. (See below for an explanation of how the Glycaemic Index works.)

As we've already said, all sorts of diets work. But we found that cutting back on carbohydrates was the most liveable-with of all the dieting options, and the least limiting in terms of losing weight while getting on with the rest of your life. When we started dieting, we followed the Atkins regime to the letter (most of the low-carb diets we have studied have a similar initial phase, where carbs are severely restricted for a minimum of a fortnight). A few weeks in, though, we started experimenting. What you are reading is the result of those experiments. We reintroduced foods in our own order. We made allowances for alcohol and chocolate. We fiddled about with existing diets and eventually, through the fiddling and through a process of trial and error, we came up with our own. We think it is more doable than many existing low-carb diets on the market – and we absolutely know, first hand, how well it works.

Here are some misconceptions about high-protein diets:

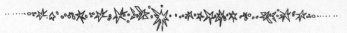

Bloody hell! My cholesterol levels are going to go through the roof!
You'll be amazed. Ours dropped quite dramatically.

What about my poor heart?
Your heart will thank you. Most high-protein diets were devised by cardiologists, and there's a reason for that: they're good for your heart. It was India's GP who encouraged her to follow a high-protein diet.

So I guzzle red meat and eggs three times a day, Atkins-style?
No. You can eat red meat, but you're going to be intelligent about it, and not wolf down insane quantities of it.

Will I have bad breath?
Yes, possibly, for a week or so. Not death-breath, or MO (for mouth odour), but a slightly weird metallic taste might appear.

Will I be horribly constipated?
Nope.

Will I feel all weak and strange? I've heard real horror stories about this way of eating.
You will feel peculiar for a maximum of five days. After that, you will feel more fantastic than you've felt in years, guaranteed. And we've all heard the horror stories. They happen because people hear about a diet like Atkins or South Beach, don't bother actually reading the book, and think they can drop all the weight they want by eating economy sausages fried in lard and triangles of processed cheese. Surprise! They can't. Double surprise: they feel like crap.

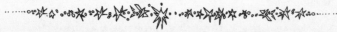

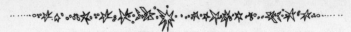

Will I eat fruit and vegetables?
Yes.

Eggs, eh? Everyone knows they're really bad for you.
Your information is out of date. From the *Daily Mail* of 19 June
2006:

Eggs have long been demonised as being bad for the heart. Yet new research suggests that this is not only untrue, but that eggs could even be considered a 'superfood'.

Eggs could actually protect against heart disease, breast cancer and eye problems and even help you to lose weight.

For years people assumed eggs were bad for cholesterol levels. But a review just published in the British Nutrition Foundation's Nutrition Bulletin found they 'have no clinically significant impact' on heart disease or cholesterol levels.

Dr Bruce Griffin of the University of Surrey's school of biomedical and molecular science analysed 30 egg studies, among them one from Harvard University which showed people who consumed one or more eggs a day were at no more risk of suffering from cardiovascular disease than non-egg eaters.

Egg yolks contain cholesterol, but nutritionists now know it is the saturated fats in food, not dietary cholesterol, that raises blood cholesterol levels, a risk factor for heart attacks.

'To view eggs solely in terms of their dietary cholesterol content is to ignore the potential benefits of eggs on coronary risk factors, including obesity and diabetes,' Dr Griffin says.

Eggs are actually good for you. 'They are rich in nutrients,' says Joanne Lunn, nutrition scientist at the British Nutrition Foundation. One egg provides 13 essential nutrients, all in the yolk (egg whites contain albumen, an important source of protein, and no fat).

Lunn says eggs are an excellent source of B vitamins, which are needed for vital functions in the body, and also provide good quantities of vitamin A, essential for normal growth and development.

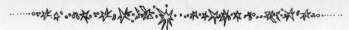

Will I never be able to have a potato, or toast, or a plate of pasta again?

Of course you will. Life's too short.

Can I drink alcohol?

Yes. Not for the first fortnight, but then yes.

What about tea and coffee?

Decaf at first, please. But then yes.

Can I have sugar?

Not for a fortnight, and then only in moderation. You can use sugar substitutes, though, if you are comfortable doing so.

What about my Diet Coke? I'm addicted to Diet Coke.

Funny, that. Everyone overweight we know – Neris included – has or had this problem. No, you're not allowed your Diet Coke. Not under any circumstances. Sorry. We'll explain later (see page 177).

But I can eat 'diet' everything else, right?

No. You absolutely cannot eat 'diet' anything. The word 'diet' means low-fat and high-carb. We don't fear (good) fat. We fear (bad) carbs. And we don't fear calories either. If you've been in the habit of counting them, forget about them right now. They're over. They play no part in this way of eating.

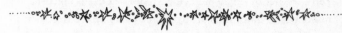

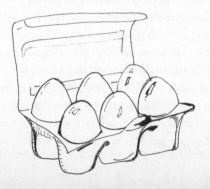

How It Works

All foods contain carbohydrates, whether you're talking about a glass of milk or about a loaf of bread. And all carbohydrates, wherever they come from, turn into sugar, or rather glucose (anything that ends in '-ose' basically means sugar – fructose from fruit, lactose from milk, etc. Bear it in mind when you're inspecting food labels). And the problem with having a lot of glucose in your system is a: that it impacts your blood-sugar levels (which is why so many of us have blood sugar 'spikes' throughout the day, when we're fine one minute and exhausted the next, until we have a bar of chocolate), and b: more crucially still, that once the sugar in your blood goes up, the pancreas kicks in and releases insulin, whose job it is to remove the sugar from your blood and get it into the cells, to be used as energy.

This is fine – unless you have so much glucose floating about that your body can't store any more. When this happens, the liver converts the glucose to fat. It doesn't tell your body to burn the fat; it tells it to store it. And hello, fat thighs.

Most of us eat too many simple carbohydrates – bread, rice, pasta, potatoes – and it thus follows that most of us have too much stored glucose, i.e. more glucose than our bodies know what to do with. This is why we're fat. In a number of cases, we may even be pre-diabetic without knowing it.

Still with us? On we go. Carbs come in two formats: complex and simple. Simple carbs are one, two or three units of sugar linked together in single molecules. Complex carbs consist of hundreds of thousands of sugar units, also linked together in single molecules. Simple sugars taste sugary, as you would expect them to. Complex carbs – potatoes, say – are not sweet. To complicate things further, complex carbs break down into two further groups: high fibre and low fibre. High-fibre carbs are difficult for us to digest, because we don't have the requisite enzyme (unlike, say, cows, which do and thus can get calories out of grass). The reason they're hard for us to digest is that they contain cellulose. But being hard to digest simply means they hang around inside our digestive tract for longer, and make our bodies work harder. It's not that we shouldn't eat them. The benefits of high-fibre foods such as broccoli or other green leafy vegetables are well known, and eating them has been associated with lowered incidences of hypertension, cancer, arthritis and diabetes.

There are no comparable benefits to low-fibre carbs, such as cereals, processed grains, pasta, potatoes or rice. Furthermore, while we know about essential fatty acids and essential amino acids, both of which are derived from protein, there is no such thing as an essential carbohydrate – i.e. it contains nothing you need that you can't get from other, non-carb foods.

For most of us, our intake of carbs comes from cereal and grain that has been processed and thus lost its fibre (just squeezing a fruit to make juice does this – processing doesn't necessarily have to involve industrial machinery. This is why, on the Glycaemic Index – see below – a mashed potato has a higher count than a whole, unpeeled boiled one).

So what we're basically doing is keeping a close and watchful eye on the simple carbs, initially by dumping them altogether. This will lighten the load both externally and when it comes to your internal organs. If you don't produce an excess of glucose, your body doesn't respond by producing an excess of insulin (which can lead to diabetes in the long term) and, crucially, your liver does not convert the glucose to fat.

Furthermore, in the absence of carbohydrates – i.e. in the absence of stored fat – your body has no choice but to start burning its own fat stores for fuel and energy. That's *your* fat, and this is why this diet works.

Eventually, you will go back to eating carbohydrates, but you will shun the processed, simple kind – the ones that made you fat in the first place. Instead, you will feast on complex carbs, which are full of fibre, vitamins, minerals and enzymes.

The first, kick-starting phase of the diet involves keeping all carbs to a minimum for a fortnight – longer if you have more than three stone to lose.

The second phase involves slowly reintroducing good

carbohydrates while still losing weight.

The third phase of the diet teaches you how to maintain your weight loss and eat a healthy, nutritious, balanced – and delicious – diet for the rest of your life. And yes, you will be allowed the odd bowl of pasta. With garlic bread on the side.

The Glycaemic Index

The Glycaemic Index measures the speed at which you digest food and convert it to glucose. As we have just seen, if you don't produce an excess of glucose, your liver does not convert the glucose to fat, because you don't give it the chance to.

The faster the food breaks down and turns to glucose, the higher the GI index, which counts sugar at 100 and compares all foods against that number.

This is pretty much all you need to know for our purposes – if you've been following this technical bit, it will come as no surprise to find, for instance, that a piece of French bread registers very highly on the GI scale, whereas a chicken breast doesn't.

And that's the boring bit over.

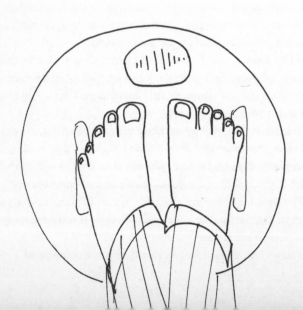

6. Are You Ready?

Good. Here come your first instructions.

Go to your local health food shop and buy the following:
▸ One good multi-vitamin without iron. Solgar (call 01442 890 355 for stockists) do an excellent one. This is to keep you nutritionally healthy while your diet is relatively limited.
▸ Psyllium husks in capsule form. These are to save you from constipation. You must take them – two in the morning.
▸ A chromium supplement containing at least 200mcg of chromium polynicotinate. Chromium builds muscle, decreases body fat and can lower cholesterol.
▸ A fish oils supplement. Because we all know they're good for you.
▸ 1000mg tablets of vitamin C if you smoke, to be taken once a day.
▸ A good vitamin B complex tablet, to be taken once a day.
▸ If you drink more than you should, you might want to give your liver a thirty-day cleanse by taking a capsule or two of Milk Thistle every day for a month.
▸ India has child-like faith in Coenzyme Q10, which boosts energy and is reputedly an anti-oxidant. I feel great when I take it (60mg daily) and less great when I don't.

Do not attempt to embark upon our diet without being armed with the above. Seriously. It won't feel good.

Have a day-long carb party. Stuff your face. Have a chip butty. Have pasta and bread. Make pancakes. Eat biscuits. Eat crisps. You get the picture. Oh, and have some milk chocolate, too. Fizzy drinks, if you like them (they sure as hell don't like you, but never mind about that for the moment).

Now clear out your kitchen. Give away the following, or put them somewhere out of reach:

▸ All your biscuits and chocolate bars.

▸ Any cold drink that isn't water.

▸ Any hot drink that isn't decaf tea or coffee, or herbal tea.

▸ Anything containing sugar (check the label – the weirdest things contain sugar, like some jarred mayonnaise, and balsamic vinegar).

▸ All pasta.

▸ All potatoes and potato-based products, including those containing potato flour (which is in many ready-meals).

▸ Anything containing wheat (i.e. flour), whether it's sweet or savoury.

▸ Any oil that isn't olive or groundnut.

▸ Any fruit (yes, we know. Fruit's supposedly good for you. But it's also full of sugar. Bear with us, it's only for two weeks).

▸ Any legumes. That means lentils, chickpeas and the like.

The kitchen's probably looking a bit tragic. Time to go shopping for the following:

▸ Meat. Any kind you like, including roasts, ham, bacon, pastrami, salami, steak, chicken, sausages (posh ones only, please – the cheap ones are full of bready fillers, and also full of crap), pâté (the good stuff that comes in slices, not the weird stuff that's like paste-in-a-tube), and so on. Check that the bacon isn't cured with sugar, and try to avoid nitrates. We strongly urge you to buy organic meat, for any number of health reasons as well as for taste ones. Yes, it's more expensive. But it tastes incomparably better.

▸ Organic free-range eggs. They have to be organic, it's non-negotiable.

▸ Fish. Any kind you like, in whatever format, from fresh seabass (which is very nice stuffed with rosemary) to canned tuna (which is very nice mixed with mayo and spring onions).

▸ Speaking of which, make sure you have either the ingredients to make your own mayonnaise, or a big fat jar of your favourite brand (but make sure it's not loaded with sugar).

▸ Olive oil and groundnut oil, if you don't have them already. Hazelnut oil makes lovely salad dressings, too.

▸ Whatever kind of vinegar you like, apart from balsamic. We like tarragon and white wine. Buy a couple of different ones if you can, to add variety to your salad dressings.

▸ Organic, additive-free peanut butter, if you like it, crunchy or smooth, but with no added sugar.

▸ Double cream (yes – double cream!).

▸ Butter (yes – butter!).

▸ New herbs and spices – if you're anything like us, chances are yours have been sitting there for some time and taste musty rather than zingy.

▸ Sea salt.

▸ Black pepper.

▸ Nuts – any kind, provided they're au naturel and with no added sugar. Don't buy the nuts yet if you have the common problem of not being able to stop eating them once you've started.

▸ Any vegetables you like, excluding potatoes, carrots, corn and peas (which are too carby for us at this stage). The best vegetables, for this diet and in general, are green, leafy ones – any kind of salad greens, any kind of spring greens, spinach, cabbages, and so on. Eat onions in moderation, i.e. use them in recipes, but don't eat three huge baked onions a day.

▸ Avocadoes, which are technically a fruit.

▸ Lemons and limes, ditto. Oh, and tomatoes.

▸ All sorts of cheeses – buffalo mozzarella, blue cheese, cheddar, brie, whatever.

▸ Mineral water, if that's your preference. We drink filtered tap water. If you don't like the idea of tap water, stock up on bottles, because water is an essential part of the diet.

▸ Whey protein powder from the health food shop. Check the carb content – some are carbier than others. Buy the lowest-carb you can find. We like Solgar (stockists from 01442 890355).

DO NOT BUY ANY LOW-CARB PRODUCTS. No bars, no shakes, nothing. They may be low-carb, but they're filled with crap, which is not what we want. You are going to be eating pure, clean food – and that means unprocessed and not crammed with odd additives.

Hopefully the larder isn't looking quite as grim by now. One last thing: keep track of your progress.

Go to www.fitday.com and open a free account. This is a marvellous tool – it's going to count your carbs for you and keep track of your weight loss. Don't worry if you don't have access to a computer, but if you do, please check it out and try to log your food intake daily.

Or just buy a journal and write down what you eat and what you feel every day. We found this an invaluable thing to do.

Okay. You're now ready to go.

▸ Weigh yourself, naked, in the morning, after you've pooed (sorry, but it does make a difference).

▸ Measure yourself if you don't know your exact height. Now get a tape measure and take these measurements (keep the tape snug, but not tight):

▸ Neck circumference

▸ Wrist circumference

▸ Bust circumference – two measurements here: one under the bosoms, along the ribcage; one where they're biggest. Waist circumference. Measure your real waist, not your low-slung jeans waist

▸ Hip circumference. Measure at the widest part.

▸ Stomach circumference. This is the measurement that made us cry, you'll be glad to hear. And no wonder: we both looked pregnant.

Write them down in this box:

Today's date is _____

I am _____ feet/metres tall _____

I weigh _____ pounds/kilos _____

My neck measures _____ centimetres/inches _____

My wrists measure centimetres/inches _____

My bust measurements are _____ and _____

My waist measurement is _____ centimetres/inches _____

My hips measure _____ centimetres/inches _____

My stomach measures _____ centimetres/inches _____

All done? We're almost ready to go. One word of caution: you
are about to embark on a life-changing way of eating. So think
about when you're going to start. Don't start dieting if you
have a wedding to go to next weekend, or if it's your birthday,
or if you have a party coming up. Don't make feeble excuses to
delay beginning, but if there's some massive social event on the
horizon, delay starting the diet until it's been and gone. There is
no point in making life unnecessarily difficult for yourself.

The first stage of the diet is the hardest. It is almost (but not
quite) identical to the first stages of Atkins, the South Beach
Diet, Protein Power and the Zone diet, among countless others.
We make no apologies for this, because this shared initial
approach demonstrably works.

It lasts a fortnight, during which you are cutting back carbs
dramatically, to between twenty and thirty grams a day. The
average-sized bowl of 'healthy' breakfast cereal contains roughly
120 grams of carbs, to give you an idea, so you're being quite
hardcore here. There are two reasons for this. 1: it works and 2:
you're taking control of your body, and of your eating, possibly
for the first time in years. That means giving it a kick up the

backside by breaking addictions to carbohydrates, primarily, but also to sugar, alcohol and caffeine.

You might feel a bit rough around the fifth day, by the way. We'd recommend timing this so that Days Five and Six are a weekend, or at least a time when you can have a little lie down. It feels a bit like coming down with the flu. We both got massive headaches on Day Five. Don't worry about it. It passes, and it doesn't come back. Much like your forthcoming weight loss, really.

The Diet, Made Simple

We're jumping the gun a bit by laying out the bare bones of the diet at this stage, but here they are. And when we say 'diet', we don't really mean 'diet'. This is more of an eating plan. For life.

Yup. We said for life.

It's okay! Don't run away! The reason it's for life is that this way of eating allows for every eventuality, *provided you stick to it in the long term*. If you do this, you can have the occasional chip butty or go on the occasional bender, and it won't affect your long-term weight loss, or weight maintenance (i.e. you won't put the pounds you've lost back on). If you stop following our method, though, the pounds *will* creep back on. This stands to reason: if you suddenly start adding two spoonfuls of sugar to every cup of tea, or scoffing half a pack of biscuits while watching telly, then you're going to get fat again. It's just a fact. A lot of diet books make all sorts of wild claims about keeping the weight off for ever. We tell it like it is. You will not put any weight back on provided you follow our plan. And if you don't, you will. Following our plan, as you will discover, is not a hardship. By the end of it, you can pretty much eat everything – though we won't lie to you and say you can go back to cereal, toast and jam at breakfast. Simple and processed carbs are no good on a daily basis (they're no good ever, actually. We don't expect you to shun them for all eternity, but we do expect you to be intelligent about them). We'll explain more in the relevant chapters. For the moment, this is what you need to know:

You are following a high-protein, low-carb diet

The absence of bad carbohydrates will mean a stop to sugar cravings, weird periods of fatigue/energy dips in the middle of the afternoon, and that general sluggish feeling you get even though you're sleeping enough. On this diet, your energy levels will rise in a way that can seem nothing short of astonishing.

You will be eating meat, fish, eggs and seafood in unlimited quantities – and quite a lot of nuts, if you like them.

These will be accessorized by lavish helpings of (mostly) green leafy vegetables for the first two weeks. We're not going down the rabbit-food route, however: your vegetables can be served with the creamiest dressings imaginable, or with lovely melted herb butters.

After the initial two weeks, your veg intake will go up considerably – we always thought we ate reasonably healthily before we embarked on this diet, but we'd never eaten as many veggies as we do now.

Eventually – after you've lost ninety per cent of the weight you want to lose – you will be eating a totally balanced diet, which will include carbohydrates, but only good ones. So, for instance, you'll be able to have your poached eggs on delicious wholemeal bread, but not on white plastic bread. Not that unbearable, is it, as a lifestyle choice?

That's it, in a nutshell: you eat lots of protein and not very many carbs. Then you gradually up the carbs, fearlessly, knowing they are 'good' carbs, which give you energy, not 'bad' carbs, which sit on your hips and make you sluggish. You also eat fat – that's good fat, like butter and olive oil, not horrible fat, like margarine (which is banned!) or 'vegetable oil'.

That's all you need to know at this stage. We'll lead you lovingly by the hand when we get to the next one.

One last thing, but it's an important one. We've said it already, but we'll just say it again. Try and eat organically wherever possible. There is no way of pretending that this doesn't make your weekly food bill more expensive, because it does. We believe the health benefits and peace of mind that come with avoiding processing, chemicals and additives are worth it. But if you are really, really hard up – we've all been there – and eating an exclusively organic diet just isn't possible, please at least try to buy organic meat. It tastes better, which is kind of crucial given how much of it you're going to consume, and it stands to reason that a battery chicken is nutritionally (to say nothing of ethically) so massively inferior to an organic one that there's really no contest. Also, when Atkins was supremely fashionable, a minority of people complained that eating the Atkins way made them feel unwell. My (India's) former neighbour was one of them, and hearing what she ate, I wasn't remotely surprised. Economy mince is not the same as ground steak. Battery chicken is not chicken. Ham made from artificially shaped 'mechanically recovered meat' is not

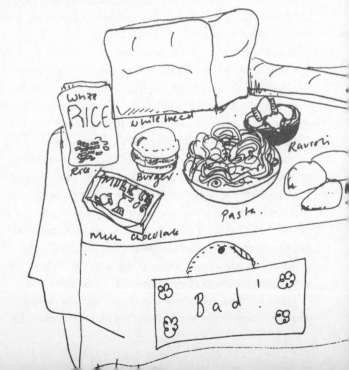

ham. Cheap sausages made of minced snout and tail and filled with (high-carb) bread and fillers are not the same as proper butchers' sausages. And plastic cheese triangles are not the same as cheese from a proper cheese shop, or even the same as a lump of decent cheddar. Please bear all of this in mind: it can make all the difference to the diet, not only in weight-loss terms, not only in health terms, but also simply in how pleasurable you find it.

On the other hand, if this simply isn't feasible, then don't worry. But do, however you choose to shop, avoid buying items that have been obviously fiddled with in some way. You want to be buying and consuming foods that are as natural and unprocessed as possible. If all else fails, buy a large, shallow terracotta pot and grow your own salad and herbs – it's incredibly easy, super-cheap in the long term, and extremely satisfying.

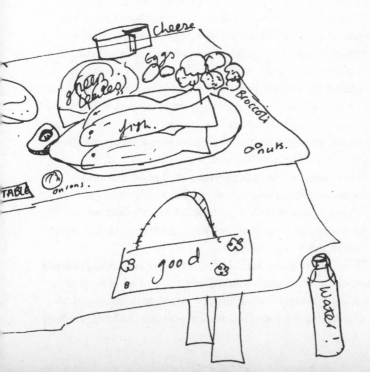

The Golden Side-Rules of Our Diet

▸ **You must drink at least eight large glasses of water a day.** This is a bare minimum. We try and aim for twelve, and fifteen wouldn't hurt. It sounds odd, and like clichéd women's-magazine stuff, but if you don't do this you will lose weight at a far slower rate than if you do. You are also more likely to be constipated, and your skin may mess up (a good side effect of this diet: really great skin). So go for it: the more water you drink, the faster you lose weight and the better you feel. Have a 1.5 litre bottle of mineral water next to you at work, and drink throughout the day. When it's gone, feel free to start (if not finish) another one. NB: when we say water, we mean water. Your minimum of eight glasses does not include herbal tea, decaf coffee or any other liquid. And that's still water, not fizzy. You can have a couple of glasses of fizzy water a day, but no more.

▸ **You absolutely must have breakfast, lunch and dinner.** On this diet, unlike on the usual calorie-controlled diets, not eating actively counts against you, and slows weight loss down. Skipping breakfast is forbidden. If your breakfast is normally a cup of coffee, train yourself gradually to broaden it out. Seriously: if you skip a meal, your weight loss will be dramatically slower than if you eat three times a day. We learned this the hard way, because it's so counter-intuitive if you're used to the old *not eating = weight loss* equation that may be familiar from low-calorie diets. You don't have to learn the truth the hard way; just do as we tell you.

▸ **It is crucial to eat a combination of good fats and protein at every meal** – so dress your salad, sauce your steak, have your prawns dunked in (preferably home-made) mayonnaise. The combination of fat and protein creates weight loss with this way of eating.

▸ **Don't make the mistake of thinking that 'dieting' means 'low-fat'.** Not in our book, it doesn't. If you try to do your own low-fat version of our diet, you won't lose the weight. If you're having three meals a day and you still feel hungry, which is possible in the early stages of the diet before your appetite re-educates itself, then for heaven's sake EAT. Have a snack. Or two, or three. Don't graze all day, obviously. But don't go hungry either.

▸ **You must have a couple of handfuls of salad leaves or other leafy green veg every day.**

▸ **You need to get off your backside at least once a day**, in a very low-tech, low-effort kind of way. We suggest walking – it's easy, everyone able-bodied can do it, and it doesn't call for any expensive equipment or gym membership. How far and how often you walk initially is up to you – but you need to begin with ten minutes a day, and walk at a pace that leaves you slightly breathless (but not chronically puffed). We're going to step this up as we progress through the diet, so you might want to invest in a pair of comfortable shoes or trainers if you don't have them already.

▸ **We'll just say it again: you really, really need to take your supplements.**

▸ **Embrace fat.** Not your own, but good, friendly fats found in delicious butter and good oils. If you like crackling, eat it. Ditto streaky bacon, or mayo, or double cream drizzled (not poured) in vegetable soup. Once again, don't, whatever you do, try to do a low-fat version of this diet, thinking it'll speed things up. It won't. It'll stall you.

▸ **Weigh yourself once a week**, after your morning poo. As the diet progresses and the weight falls off, the temptation to jump on the scales five times a day is overwhelming. Try to resist it. Weight loss is not linear: your weight fluctuates fairly wildly even as you're losing it, and if you suddenly find yourself two pounds heavier today than you were yesterday, you'll get depressed – even though it all evens out in the end. So aim for once a week, and ignore the scales, or avoid them altogether, before and during your period.

▸ **Use a tape measure as well as the scales.** I (India) lost two inches off my waist before I lost a single pound. Mysterious. Again, don't measure yourself every day. Twice a week, tops.

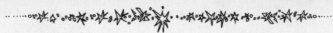

The recipes given for the next fortnight are interchangeable. If you don't fancy the suggestions on any given day, skip forwards or backwards for other ideas – or ignore them altogether and substitute your own favourites. And please bear in mind that the recipes we're giving are for things we like to eat. You don't have to make any of them if you don't want to! They're here as guidance only. Any cookbook will contain recipes for things you can eat, and if you're a keen cook, you can make things up and adjust methods as you go along, substituting parmesan for bread crumbs, for instance, or, in some cases (and later on in the diet), ground almonds for flour.

If you need more recipes, or further ideas, or if the idea of adjusting existing recipes makes you feel nervous, we strongly recommend the two following cookbooks, which are specifically low-carb, and which you can therefore cook from with impunity, knowing you're not sneaking in any forbidden ingredients:

The Low-Carb Gourmet by Karen Barnaby. Published by Rodale International Ltd, price £12.99, ISBN: 1405087935.

There are an awful lot of low-carb cookbooks around, but a lot of them don't really float our boat. This one is wonderful, and written with passion. We've not cooked a duff recipe from it yet.

The Low-Carb Cookbook by Fran McCullough, published in the US by Hyperion, price $23.99 (you'll have to get your bookshop to order this – we think it's worth it. The ISBN they'll need is 0786862734. Or order from amazon.com).

Extremely comprehensive, imaginative, glorious – a kitchen bible, really.

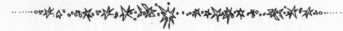

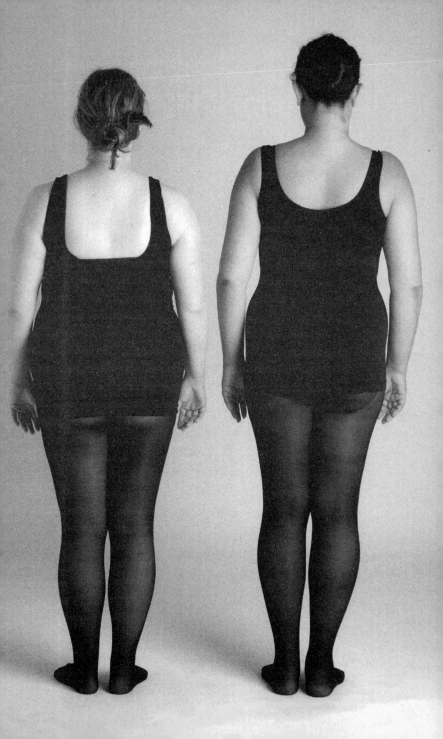

Part Two
The Diet – Phase One

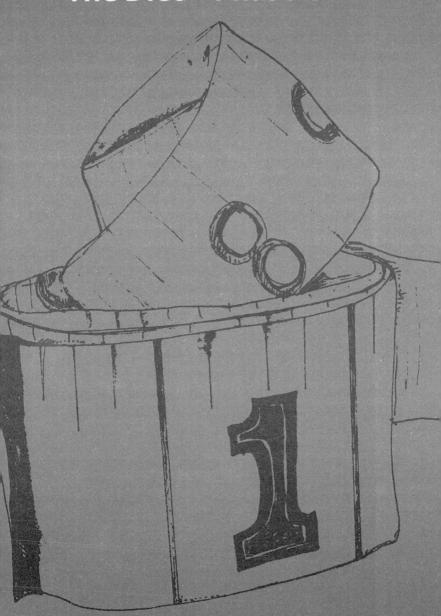

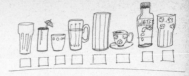

Phase One Day One

Oakey-pokey. Here we go: Good morning! And welcome to the first day of the new you.

Before you even get out of bed, realize this: you are NEVER AGAIN going to be as fat as you are today. Weight-wise, it's downhill all the way from here. Today, you are the fattest you're ever going to be.

So that's quite a nice thought, isn't it?

You can get up now, and go to the kitchen. If it's at all possible, feed your family before you feed yourself, or get up a bit earlier and feed yourself before you feed them. Or tell them to feed themselves, the lazy sods (unless they're infants, in which case, aaaah). You're only going to do this for a couple of days, while you get into the swing of things – afterwards, you'll all be eating at the same time. For now, though, ease yourself in.

Anyway, try and find the time for breakfast. Grabbing things on the hoof is not allowed. Sit down, please, in as calm an environment as possible, and use cutlery. Do not read the paper while you're eating. Do not put the telly on. Concentrate on what you're doing. If you are rushing out the door to the office on an empty stomach – STOP! Eat your breakfast first.

First Things First

Pour yourself a large glass of water, sip some, take your supplements, and drink up the rest. Have another glass of water if you can bear it. (Before you ask, yes, you are going to be peeing a lot for the first few days.)

This is why we're going to keep telling you to drink a great deal of water:

▸ Water suppresses the appetite.
▸ Water helps the body to metabolize fat.
▸ Your kidneys can't function properly if you're dehydrated
– and you're already dehydrated by the time you feel thirsty.

- If your kidneys can't cope, your liver helps out. This distracts it from one of its normal jobs, which is to metabolize stored fat to use as energy. If it can't do this, you don't lose weight.
- Water is the best antidote to fluid retention.
- Water helps maintain muscle tone by keeping muscles hydrated.
- Water helps to flush out waste.
- It regulates body temperature.
- It protects your organs and tissues.

So, when we say drink your water, we really, REALLY mean it. Not just because of anecdotal evidence, but because we know for ourselves that if you don't drink enough, you don't lose enough – plus you feel like crap. Just do it.

Breakfast

Today, it's bacon and eggs. If you don't fancy bacon and eggs, flip forward a day or two for other suggestions. But let's assume you find bacon and eggs delicious (who doesn't, really?).

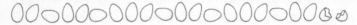

2 eggs
4 rashers of bacon
freshly ground black pepper

Fry the whole lot up in a dash of groundnut oil. You can have a handful of mushrooms fried in butter on the side, and half a tomato, if you like.

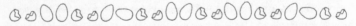

You can drink decaffeinated tea or coffee, but with cream rather than milk. Or try any kind of unsweetened herbal tea. I (India) used to have a heaped teaspoon of sugar in my tea every morning (and on about twenty other occasions throughout the day). Going without it felt weird for a couple of days. Now, if I'm given sweet tea by accident, it tastes so nauseating I want to spit it out.

Useful Tip

Rooibos tea is wonderful. It's organic and caffeine-free, full of anti-oxidants, and incredibly good for you, plus it tastes yummy. The trick is to leave the bag in the water for at least four minutes (or more – it doesn't 'stew' like ordinary tea). It's good for everything from skin to sinuses, and more satisfying than ordinary herbal tea. Also, it makes you feel like a Number 1 Lady Detective. Ow!

Neris takes her decaf tea bags to work and keeps them in her desk drawer. She can't tell the difference between them and normal tea.

Have as many cups of decaf tea/coffee/herbal tea as you like during the course of today.

In a few days' time, you may find that post-breakfast is automatic pooing time. This is very good. Always weigh yourself after you poo, please – grotesquely enough, it does make a difference. Also, in time you'll notice that your poos stop being offensive. If you had any issues with wind (oh dear, what hideous nitty-gritty, and it's only Day One), they will disappear. If you had inconsistent bowel movements (varying from day to day), this too will, er, pass. You end up with incredibly efficient superpoos that just happen, are comparatively odourless, and require a mere couple of sheets of loo paper to deal with. Sorry if that's too much information, but this really isn't the place to be coy.

Find the time, between now and lunch, to go for a walk. We're talking ten minutes, but briskly. Get off the Tube one stop early and walk the rest of the way, or walk round your garden a few times, or round the block, or whatever. You want to break into a light sweat, but not be so puffed that you're practically jogging. Reward yourself with another large glass of water or two. If you're peckish, have any of the snacks allowed.

Lunch

Today, try one of these:

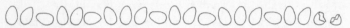

STEAK AU POIVRE

Easy way: have it in a restaurant, with a side salad. Marginally less easy way: make it yourself.

ONE STEAK
peppercorns
butter
double cream

SALAD INGREDIENTS
avocado
blue cheese dressing (recipe on page 90)

Get a pestle and mortar or clean coffee grinder and crush a small handful of black peppercorns. Melt a knob of butter in a pan. Press the peppercorns into both sides of the steak so they stick. When the butter sizzles, add the steak and turn up the heat to medium.

Toss yourself a small salad while it's cooking. Put some avocado in it. Have blue cheese dressing if you wish.

Flip the steak over after a couple of minutes. It should be nice and crusty on one side. To test, poke the middle of the steak firmly with a finger. Springy – rare; less springy – medium; firm – well done.

Remove to a plate. Pour a glug of double cream into the buttery/steaky juice, let it bubble for a couple of seconds, then pour on to the waiting steak.

Eat. And don't forget to drink your water, too.

SALADE NICOISE

Ditto about the restaurant or café. Otherwise, mix together the following:

salad leaves of your choice
half a tomato, chopped up small
1 can of tuna in olive oil
a handful of cooked green beans
a couple of hard boiled eggs, each cut into four or six 'crescents'
flat leaf parsley

sea salt and black pepper
vinaigrette (recipe on page 90)

Jumble it all together.
   Eat.

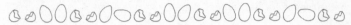

If you're still hungry, have more. If you're still hungry, have a plate of cheese.

   Now carry on with your afternoon.

Supper

If you like olives or nuts, nibble on a handful while you're cooking. Have a glass of water while you're at it.

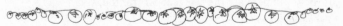

CAULIFLOWER FAUX-MASH

We used to HATE cauliflower. Now, to us, cauliflower rocks. Please try this – it's fantastic.

half a cauliflower
butter
double cream
salt and pepper
nutmeg, if you like

Steam the cauliflower florets until very tender. Chuck into a blender. Blend with a generous knob of butter and a glug of cream. Season. Serve. (Use any leftovers for fried mash cakes for tomorrow's breakfast.)

 Tip: faux-mash makes an excellent topping for this diet's version of shepherd's pie, or cottage pie (see recipe page 115), and works as a substitute wherever you would ordinarily use mash.

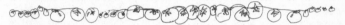

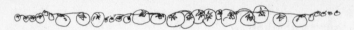

TARRAGON CHICKEN

1 organic chicken breast per person, more if you're starving
1 bunch of fresh tarragon
1 small pot of double cream
butter
groundnut oil
half a lemon

Cut the chicken into strips, or chunks if you prefer. Melt the butter in the pan on medium heat and add a tiny blob of groundnut oil. When it's sizzling, add the tarragon and chicken strips, and cook the strips until they go crispy and brown (if crispy and brown and a bit sticky is what you like. I know I do). Add enough cream to make a sauce – a third to half of the small tub should do it. Wait a minute for it all to meld and bubble. Add the juice from the lemon, taste, and season if you think it needs it. Eat with the mash. Drink your water.

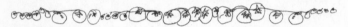

That wasn't so hard, was it? And pretty delicious, if we say so ourselves. Give yourself a pat on the back, my friend – you've made it through Day One.

Thought for the Day

Obstacles are what you see if you take your eyes off the goal.

How We Felt on Day One

It doesn't feel much like a diet.

Here is more of what we thought when we were in your shoes, just starting out. We kept journals throughout our diet journey, and here are the relevant bits for today.

India: *I am just under sixteen stone. For God's sake.*

Not sure I'm doing this diet right – feel like I haven't stopped eating. Don't feel remotely hungry. Well, I did feel hungry every now and then, so I ate. Not sure about sugarless tea, but hey, there are worse things. What's different is that today I had that boring thing

that nutritionists always talk about: Three Proper Meals. Usually I just graze constantly.

Must have had a lot of calories. Ah well. I have faith. Well, kind of . . . I can't get over how much I ate. Had salami for snacks, and olives. So much fat. Good fat, though – olive oil and butter.

Quite weird having nothing sweet at all. Don't have sweet tooth, so not too bad, but I'd be unhappy if I were a chocoholic.

Peed loads. Like being eight months pregnant.

Feel very gung-ho, though. Quite excited. My main thought so far is: this is painless. Actually, forget excited – am exhilarated by the possibilities.

Neris: *It's Day One and I weigh sixteen stone ten pounds.*

Have got to do this. This has to be the last diet I ever go on. I've got to try to stick to it.

If ever there was a sign that I should be doing this it must be the three people who stopped me yesterday:

10.00am: The bank manager said to me in the bank today, 'Mrs Johnson, obviously with the imminent arrival there will be a lot of changes for you so we should talk about some saving schemes!' Stunned. I'm afraid I went along with him. I could not be bothered to argue and just said, 'Yes it is going to be really busy. I won't be able to talk to you for a few months, until it has all settled down again.' What a cheek. Does it look that obvious?

Having never had a full-length mirror I have not had the time since my daughter was born (over two years ago!) to really think about the stark reality of what I actually look like. I know I have been a bit silly and kept wearing some of my stretchy maternity clothes. I know that is uncool and it is not something I am proud of.

Anyway, at 11.30 (this is not an exaggeration) I told the woman in the local clothes shop that I was about to go on a diet. She replied, 'Is that healthy when you are so far gone?' There followed a 3pm encounter with a woman I know (vaguely) who crossed the street to congratulate me on my bump. After these three incidents I thought it was all funny but I did feel slightly empty. I'm not joking but that really was all in one day.

So there you go. I've got to do this. I have spent years and years doing diets where I fixate about a date in the future, like a wedding, a birthday or a party, and I just go all out for that but then I lose my momentum. I need to change things long term now. I don't have the energy for anything else. So off I go.

Pm. I have a throbbing head. I feel like my shoulders weigh a ton. And I'm very, very bleary. But hurrah I've stuck to it.

I've had decaf tea, three eggs scrambled with two tablespoons of double cream and a blob of butter.

My lovely lunch left me strangely full: I got a salade nicoise from the sandwich bar around the corner from work. Hurrah. For dinner I made a huge effort making the Chicken Tarragon. I'm a rubbish cook but India assured me it was easy, and it was. And really nice to eat.

Felt really pleased with myself, like I'd achieved something.

I drank so much water and decaf tea. I'm on the toilet a lot which is a bit annoying but I feel quite good.

It's easy to stick to the food. I'm on a roll but don't expect me to be interesting. My head hurts too much.

I'm going to do it this time.

Staple recipes of the day

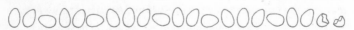

BLUE CHEESE DRESSING
Blend 1 cup mayo with 1 cup sour cream. Add enough olive oil to make it dressing consistency. Season. Add a good handful of crumbled blue cheese.

VINAIGRETTE
In a clean jam jar, put one third vinegar (not balsamic) to two–thirds olive oil. Add lemon juice or mustard to taste. Season. Put the lid on and give it a shake. That's it. Add garlic, herbs or both for variety.

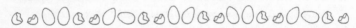

Phase One Day Two

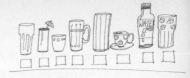

Good morning! We hope you're feeling good and full of optimism. You're also probably feeling slightly strange. This is absolutely normal. Work with it. Stick at it. It will pass. Not only are you losing weight, but you're also detoxing. Your body needs to catch up with itself, and when it does, it's going to be very, very happy, and reward you with some serious and dramatic shrinkage.

Before we start today, we'd like you to congratulate yourself on having made it through yesterday. The beginning of the diet is the hardest part, and you're on the way.

Like yesterday, and like every day in the future, yea, even until the end of time, start by taking your supplements and drinking a big glass of water, or two if you can manage it. You're allowed a slice of lemon or lime in there, if you like, for a bit of added zing.

Breakfast

Eventually, you're going to re-educate your taste buds so that certain foods that you don't traditionally think of as 'breakfasty' become part of your eating regime. For the moment, though, let's stick to the more traditional options. You're welcome to have bacon and eggs again, but let's say today you fancy sausages. Fry or grill them using butter or groundnut oil. Remember, if the former, to add a dot of oil to the butter to stop it from burning – this is always necessary when frying in butter, unless you deliberately want the nutty taste of 'burnt' butter. Accessorize with half a grilled tomato. Chuck in an egg if you fancy it, and/or a handful of mushrooms. If you have any cauliflower mash left over from yesterday, fry it up into cakes.

Eat sitting down, and with cutlery. Drink some water – before or after the meal, ideally, so that everything isn't sloshing about in your stomach like soup.

Do whatever you do in the morning (in our case, resist the fairly overwhelming urge to go back to bed, and try to get on with work instead). Mid-morning, if that's convenient, go for a little walk. Yesterday's was ten minutes. It would be good if today's was fifteen, if that's manageable. If not, then ten is fine. Remember: you want to be slightly out of breath, but not huffing and puffing.

Lunch

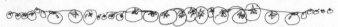

ROAST BUTTERNUT SQUASH SOUP WITH PARMESAN AND BACON
Piece of cake, this (well, not quite cake), and delicious.

one butternut squash
olive oil
vegetable or chicken stock (cubes are fine, Marigold is better)
Parmesan cheese, grated
crispy bacon

Cut the butternut squash in two lengthways. Brush it with olive oil and stick it in the oven, heated to 190°C, gas 5, for an hour or so, depending on its size – it's ready when soft. Scoop out the flesh and whizz it in a blender. Put it in a pan with enough vegetable or chicken stock to achieve a consistency that's pleasing to you. Gently heat through for twenty minutes or so. Serve with one big heaped tablespoon of Parmesan per bowl, and some crispy, crumbled bacon. Feel free to have seconds.

If you want to gild the lily, you could add some rosemary leaves to the roasting squash, and/or drizzle the finished product with a little truffle oil.

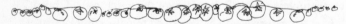

If you're still hungry, have a side salad – not a gigantic, main-course size one, but a couple of handfuls of leaves, dressed however you like (excepting, of course, any sugary dressing). Good olive oil and lemon juice make a lovely, crisp dressing which is quite nice after the richness of the soup. Have a piece of cheese if you're still hungry.

This is all very lovely, but I work in an office. What do I eat?
You bring a packed lunch, or go out to your local sandwich bar.
A packed lunch isn't terribly glamorous, granted, but at least you
know exactly what's in it, which in the circumstances is extremely
helpful. The problem with ready-made stuff is that so much of
it contains hidden carbs, and also often hidden sugars. Most of
the recipes in this book can be slung into some Tupperware and
reheated, if your office should run to a microwave.

Failing that, though, what you're after – apart from lunch on
expenses, because as you'll already be able to see, this diet is
extremely restaurant-friendly – is an old-fashioned sandwich
shop, of the kind that has sandwich fillings laid out in boxes
behind a glass counter. If you should be lucky enough to be within
striking distance of such a gem, cherish it and make friends with
the staff. Have a recce, and then choose from any of the following
breadless options. Have generous dollops of any of the following:

▶ prawn mayonnaise
▶ egg mayonnaise
▶ tuna mayonnaise (there's a bit of a theme developing here)
▶ crispy bacon
▶ sliced tomato
▶ sliced cucumber
▶ sliced avocado
▶ sliced olives
▶ smoked salmon
▶ cream cheese
▶ any other kind of cheese – mozzarella is nice with tomato
and avocado
▶ roast beef (and you can have horseradish with it)[3]
▶ roast pork, lamb, etc.
▶ hams
▶ any fish

---

[3] Horseradish seems to speed up weight loss for some people. We don't know why. If you like
roast beef, try and have creamed horseradish on the side.

- salamis and other cold meats
- sausages
- pâté
- taramasalata, if it's not bulked out with bread (ask)

Ask for any of these ingredients in salad form, i.e. with lettuce and dressing (check for sugar), or have the salad on the side and use the lettuce to make wraps. It's not necessarily wildly exciting, but then neither is it significantly more boring than the usual lunchtime sarnie, frankly.

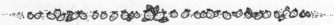

Get on with your afternoon, and remember – if you're hungry, eat. Have some nuts in your bag, like a squirrel. And please remember to keep drinking your water, along with any decaf tea/coffee you might fancy.

Supper

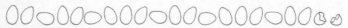

ROAST COD WITH HERBS AND TOMATOES; SIDE SALAD

1 cod fillet per person – two if you're starving
good olive oil
half a tomato per person, sliced
generous handful of any fresh herb, or mixture of fresh herbs, if you like
  – try thyme and rosemary

Brush each cod fillet – and it doesn't have to be cod, it could be any other robust and fresh-looking fish – with olive oil. Cover with sliced tomato. Crush the herbs a little so they release their fragrance, and stick them on top of the cod. Wrap the whole thing up neatly – or messily, if you must – in tin foil. Roast at 190°C, gas 5, for fifteen minutes. Serve. Don't forget to pour the herby olive oil that's puddled at the bottom of the foil on to the fish. Serve with a salad – it's nice with rocket and Parmesan.

You'll notice we're low on puddings. That is because one of us (India) disapproves of artificial sweeteners, especially at this stage of the diet, when you're weaning yourself off sugar. But don't worry – we'll go into your pudding options in a few days, though they are limited.

Drink your water.

Useful Tip
Make herb butters to melt on to meat or fish. Let unsalted butter soften at room temperature and add chopped fresh herbs; shape into a roll using cling film; refrigerate. Then cut off a slice or two to melt on to your steak (or whatever). You can make garlic butter this way too, and blue cheese and walnut, which is especially nice with beef.

Thought for the Day
If I can repeat failure, I can repeat success.

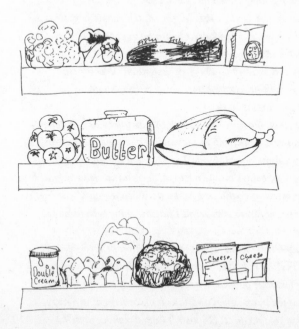

How We Felt on Day Two

India: *I still feel gung-ho. I also feel odd in a way that's hard to describe: I'm perfectly fine, and functioning normally, but I feel a bit speedy and there's a weird (not bad, just weird) taste in my mouth. I keep brushing my teeth. All of this so far is fine, except that earlier I really wanted a Starbucks vanilla latte, for some peculiar reason – I normally have them about twice a month. Milk aside, I don't think sugary syrup is really an option. Bummer. Never mind. Went to a restaurant for dinner. Odd to have no wine. Ate a fillet steak with béarnaise sauce and a side of creamed spinach (yummy), and then a cheese plate. Felt oddly indifferent to the bread on the table. Wonder how long that'll last.*

Was lovely to come home a: sober (not that I make a habit of getting pissed! I just mean it was nice to be clear-headed and not even a tiny bit tiddly), and b: not stuffed, but – horrible phrase – 'pleasantly full'. Just as well, as the baby was up in the night.

Told someone I was following a high-protein diet. She was delighted to tell me some ridiculous story about a woman a friend of a friend knows. For God's sake. Might not tell people I'm dieting. They're weirdly keen to come forward with horror stories. Sisterhood, eh?

I haven't pooed since the day before yesterday, which doesn't feel great. Very slight headache before going to bed (in about two minutes), but am hoping to sleep it off.

On the plus side, though: I'm finding this diet very easy to follow. I don't have a sweet tooth, so I'm not missing the sugar (except in my tea and hypothetical latte), and I really liked the fact that I could have eaten loads of things on the menu at the restaurant. Very glad I didn't have to interrogate the waiter at length about ingredients – it's all very obvious. So far, so good. And I haven't once been hungry.

Neris: *Woke up feeling like I've got mild flu. Drowsy, irritable and blocked nose. Feeling rubbish, basically. Couldn't help but weigh myself. Wow – lost four pounds! My body is so weird. I can literally put on five pounds in one meal and take it off overnight. Anyway, still going to keep going on it. (I mustn't keep weighing myself.)*

Don't understand how the weight actually disappears . . . but it has gone.

Had some bacon and scrambled eggs for breakfast. It's 11.08 now and I feel really full. Which is also extraordinary for me!

I did have one chunk of cheese ten minutes ago, though, which should keep me going until lunch. Desperately need a Twix bar. Life would be so nice if I could just eat one with a nice cup of normal tea.

5pm. Feeling rubbish. Sluggish. Overwhelmingly tired. If I closed my eyes now I would go to sleep (not good when I'm supposed to go in to a meeting in about five minutes). I feel a bit embarrassed by how much I'd like to go off the diet already and its only Day Two. You really have to be focused and have an excuse to go off it. Then I see myself in the mirror or look at a shop full of millions of items of clothes that I could never fit – it is those moments when I really feel angry with myself – the rest of the time I sort of feel normal and don't see why I can't eat what I want. Then I feel angry with myself that I got into this situation and that I've wasted so much time trying to just get rid of this weight. Feeling this rubbish and fluey doesn't help the general downward spiral. Went to bed feeling not at all hungry.

Haven't drunk enough water. Only had a litre. Every time I had water through the day I felt better, though, so I'm going to try to have more tomorrow. Finding it difficult working and feeling a bit rough.

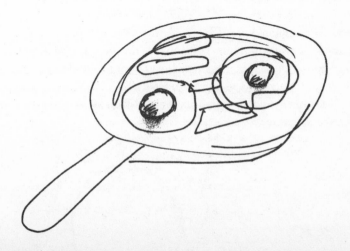

Phase One Day Three

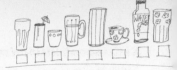

Well, we're very happy to see you still with us. You are very possibly not feeling that fabulous today. Or maybe you are: Neris was practically a wreck on the third day, and I was pretty much fine. Some people are fortunate enough to go through this early stage of the diet feeling A-okay, and some (the majority, I would say) find they have a couple of rather rough days. All we can say, now we're ten stone down, is please bear with us. And if you're feeling wonderful, please don't panic and convince yourself you're going to feel dreadful tomorrow, because it's not by any means a given. I think that perhaps I felt better than Neris because I didn't eat very much sugar (or chocolate which is Neris's thing) before the diet, so the lack of it was less of a shock to my system. But maybe that had nothing to do with it at all. The point is, it'll pass. Any day now, you're going to wake up feeling unusually fantastic. We promise.

So: you should be reasonably familiar with the morning drill by now. Take your supplements. Drink your water, and have another glass if you can manage it.

Breakfast

This morning, as a change from eggs, we're going to have smoked salmon and cream cheese. Buy some smoked salmon. Buy a tub of cream cheese – the genuine article, please, not any 'light' version. Spread the cream cheese generously on any number of pieces of smoked salmon, roll up and eat, with lemon juice and black pepper if you like. If you want to add sliced avocado to your roll-ups, go right ahead.

Remember to go for your walk. We're still on fifteen minutes if you can manage it.

A Little Look Inside Your Closet

Today, we're going to go off at a slight tangent and give you an additional project. We want you to have a really good look at your wardrobe. If you're anything like us, it contains a load of garments that are only in there not because they're gorgeous, not because they make you feel fabulous, but because they fit. We've all done that kind of panicky shopping, grabbing the nearest black sack because it isn't eye-bleedingly ugly, and it's got enough Lycra in it to cover a multitude of sins.

Soon – sooner than you imagine, if you stick at it – you are going to have to acquire a whole new wardrobe. There's an entire chapter on dressing for your size coming up, but for the moment we need you to do the following:

Equip yourself with some bin bags.

If you have breasts larger than a 34C, put any round-necked tops, polo necks or T-shirts in the bin bag. You don't have to throw them away: just store them somewhere for the time being. On the other hand, if you're confident with a pair of scissors, you can cut the T-shirts into V-necks.

Put anything with an elasticated waist into the bin bag, excepting pyjamas or tracky bottoms. Elasticated waists do nothing for anyone and not having any waistbands digging into you only encourages you to pretend you don't have a weight problem.

Have a look in the mirror and work out what the widest part of your body is. It is likely to be your stomach or your backside. Now chuck out any item of clothing that ends where your widest part begins: tops that end just above the bottom; shirts that end where your stomach starts.

Put aside anything bulky, unless it's very cold outside and you have no central heating. Those classic items of comfort wear – big sweatshirts, thick, loose sweaters, baggy shirts – do nobody any favours. Get rid of them.

If you have any leggings lurking around, throw them out if you're over thirty, unless you can genuinely state that you have spectacular legs. Even if you do, beware of leggings that end at the widest part of your calf.

Skirts: if they're in any way gathered or pleated, chuck them out. Any extra fabric around the stomach is a disaster, and makes you look twice as wide as you already are. Basically, bulk makes you bulky. We're not suggesting you totter about in pencil skirts, but a narrow silhouette is what you're after, so anything floaty, 'peasanty', pleated or bunchy is a no-no. You want a really clean line, and no centre fastenings, i.e. buttons around the stomach. A hook-and-eye fastening to the side of your waist is best.

Trousers: be brutal with yourself. If they're skin-tight on the thighs, dump them (unless you're the Leggings Queen with the spectacular legs). If they're skin-tight across the butt, ditto. Be very, very careful with jeans, which can add an extraordinary amount of bulk if they're badly cut, as most are. The pleated rule above applies here, too – even more so, in fact – there is nothing – nothing – less flattering to a full figure than pleated, chino-style trousers.

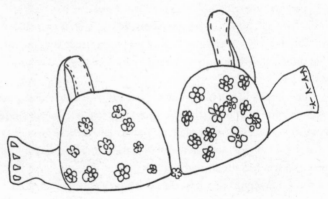

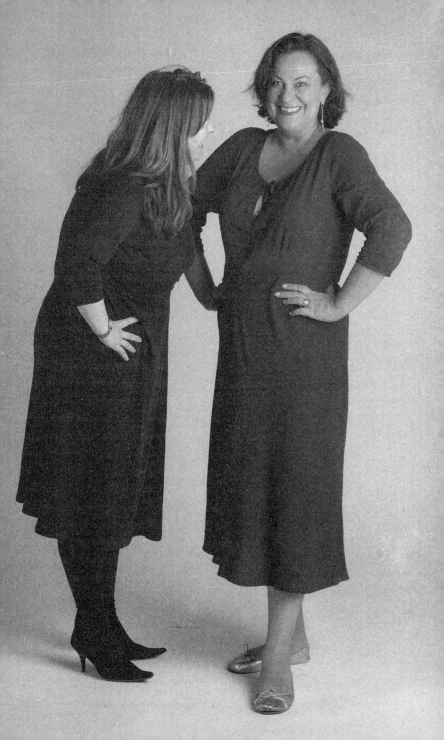

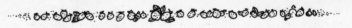

So what can I wear?

What you are after are thin, relatively fitted clothes. Not only are these the most flattering things to wear when you're carrying extra bulk, but they can be layered to great effect. So, dig out tea dresses, thin, form-skimming (but not tight), U-necked or V-necked cotton tops, unbulky jerseys and cardigans, tunic tops. These will form the staple of your wardrobe for the next few weeks. It is a myth that if you are fat you need to swamp yourself in loose tent-like garments: these simply make you look like an unlovely cross between Demis Roussos and Big Daddy. We don't understand why shops persist in selling them, and in urging you towards them if you're a size eighteen or above. They're hideous. Neris wrote in her diary: 'I looked at my clothes and realized they consisted of my "fat" wardrobe (going up to size twenty-four and then some maternity stuff that I still occasionally wear) and my 'thin' wardrobe (a couple of foxy size twelve suits both worn only once in 1999) and all the sizes in between. I have put everything that didn't fit me ON THIS VERY DAY into plastic bags, labelled them by size and put them in the drawers under the bed. For the first time I can actually see the choice of clothes I REALLY HAVE. And realize all I have is fifteen different types of black top and actually not much apart from that.'

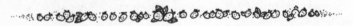

On pages 190–3 you will find tips for looking the best you can at all stage of weight loss. For the time being, it's only Day Three, and we just want you to have a think about the future. As far as dressing for now is concerned, try to remember the following simple rules:

Wrap dresses actually actively look better on curves than they do on skinny bodies. They must be the right size, though – having a gaping band of material where the 'wrap' bit of fabric has been yanked too tight looks (and feels) horrible. Every high street store stocks wrap dresses, which have become classics. Wear with a pretty camisole underneath for work, and with a beautiful necklace and some cleavage for the evening.

Reasonably tailored clothes are more flattering than shapeless sacks, even if a shapeless sack is exactly what you feel like. You need a proper waistband, too.

You're never too fat for **pretty tights or stockings,** or for pretty shoes. Don't slob about in comfy flatties all the time: a small heel dramatically improves anybody's legs, and patterned hosiery draws attention away from a hefty mid-section. We love fishnets, but again, your local department store will leave you spoilt for choice.

Scoop necks or V-necks win out over high necks every time.

Invest in some control pants. They're not by any stretch of the imagination a lovely garment, but they absolutely work. Marks and Spencer's Magic Knickers are, we believe, an absolutely essential piece of kit.

Go and get measured for a bra, if you didn't heed our advice earlier in this book. The majority of British women wear the wrong size, and a well-fitting bra can make all the difference to the appearance of your chest. If you're fat, the last thing you need is a bra that creates strange rolls of blubber by your armpits, or one that bisects your bosoms so that you appear to have four instead of two. Also, if you don't have enough uplift from your bra, your chest appears to meld seamlessly into your stomach, which is a really, really bad look, and one that is sadly

very common in overweight women. We recommend Rigby
& Peller, Bravissimo, John Lewis and M&S as good places to
get fitted.

Wear nothing sausage-tight, but wear nothing ridiculously
loose either.

Accessorize like mad, and get in touch with your
inner makeup artist. It might be an idea to have a series of
department store makeovers over the next couple of weeks
– but do your homework: if the woman approaching you with
her brushes and lipsticks has an orange face and stripes of
burgundy blusher, go elsewhere.

Underwear aside, if our recommendations entail a shopping
trip because you have nothing resembling the clothes we
suggest, please don't go mad, and please only buy cheap things
– we like H&M, whose range goes up to a size thirty, and New
Look, whose range goes up to size twenty-four. The clothes
you buy now will be too big in a matter of weeks, so don't go
overboard.

That's probably enough to be getting on with. Incidentally,
by Day Three you may very well find that some parts of your
clothing – the waistband, or across the shoulders, or over
the bust – feel looser. This is why we're suggesting thinking
about your wardrobe. You are probably feeling a mixture of
apprehension and excitement at the weeks ahead, and we have
found that thinking about clothes – particularly about the
sorts of clothes we wouldn't have dreamed of wearing when we
started, like titchy designer jeans – was an excellent incentive.
Because the truth of the matter is that, no matter how fat you
feel now, you're shrinking. And if you want designer jeans,
my dears, you shall have them – and look fabulous in them.
But not quite yet.

Lunch

We're assuming you've been busy with the bin bags and that
there isn't really any time to cook today. Have an omelette – it's
delicious, it's filling, and it takes minutes to make. Choose from

any of the allowed fillings – cheese, or a combination of cheeses, green leafy veg, tomatoes, onions, garlic, ham, salami, cold meats, and so on. Or go the whole hog and make a big Spanish omelette, which you can cut into chunks and help yourself to throughout the day. Drink your water.

Supper

One of the pleasing things about our diet is that it is so supremely restaurant-friendly. Tonight, we suggest you find this out for yourself, either by venturing out or by ordering a takeaway. I (India) eat industrial amounts of Indian food, which fits in with this way of eating beautifully. No rice or bread, obviously, and no mango chutney – though you're allowed pickles. Most South Indian food, with its reliance on pancakes and batter, is out for the time being, but anything else is more than allowed. Grilled meats, like lamb kebabs or chicken tikka, are made for this diet. Creamy curries, provided they contain no potato, are heaven-sent, and vegetable curries are a brilliant way of getting your greens. Chinese food is another possibility: crispy duck (and a dollop of plum sauce isn't going to kill you just this once, provided you don't make a daily habit of it), braised meats, steamed fish or seafood, all those sizzling dishes, and of course bok choi, a fantastic choice as far as green leafy veg are concerned. If you like Japanese food, go mad with the sashimi. Here are some other diet-friendly restaurant foods:

- ▶ chicken satay
- ▶ seabass with ginger and spring onions
- ▶ roast duck
- ▶ chicken liver pâté
- ▶ smoked salmon in all its manifestations
- ▶ mozzarella, basil and tomato salad
- ▶ omelettes (if you haven't had one for lunch)
- ▶ grilled meats
- ▶ liver and onions
- ▶ roast meats, e.g. roast pork and crackling, or roast chicken

- kebabs
- eggs Benedict or Florentine, without the muffin but with lots of hollandaise
- Caesar salad, minus the croutons
- most soups
- pretty much any fish dish you care to mention
- lobster, langoustines and crab
- antipasti – salami, cheese, olives
- beef or tuna carpaccio
- ceviche
- fruits de mer
- osso bucco
- moules marinières
- chateaubriand with béarnaise sauce
- sauerkraut
- oysters

And that's only the tip of a pretty massive iceberg.

Thought for the Day
Believe in yourself. You can do it.

How We Felt on Day Three
India: *I'm in the swing now. I can totally do this – to my amazement, I don't find any aspect of this diet difficult. Even my sugarless tea was much more bearable today. Marched briskly around the park for fifteen minutes – tremendously boring, especially as it was drizzling. Face went bright red, and of course I bumped into two people I knew, looking deeply unphotogenic, with crimson face and frizzy rain-hair. Went to a drinks party tonight, which would have been a great deal more fun if I could have had a drink, but am determined not to drink for at least a fortnight (famous last words). Being totally sober in a room filled with drunken people is boring in the extreme. Left after half an hour and was home by 8.30, which I took great pleasure in – a week ago I'd have stayed longer, got mildly drunk by accident, come home late, fallen into bed and woken up feeling a bit rough.*

As it was, had a bath and watched telly in bed, feeling very smug and pleased with myself.

Emailed Dr S, my GP, to ask him what he thought of the whole high-protein/low-carb thing. He was extremely encouraging and in favour. I might have some blood tests done, to compare and contrast before and after. I DO still feel peculiar, but it's manageable. Low-level headache.

There is quite a peculiar taste in my mouth, but I'm getting used to it. Paranoid about halitosis, though A, whom I breathe on like a dragon, assures me this isn't the case. Still, though – go out and buy a Sonicare toothbrush and industrial quantities of floss. Later, discover to my horror that meat has a horrible way of lodging itself between your teeth and, uh, decaying. Am now going to floss and brush after every meal.

Didn't poo today. I really hate not pooing. I hope there's some poo-action tomorrow.

Neris: *Stayed same weight (I did weigh. Sorry). Shouldn't have but couldn't resist. But found myself deflated by not having lost weight. Really don't want to do that again. Exhausted again. But to be honest I'm always exhausted, ever since having my daughter (maybe even before if I'm honest). Feel like I've got something wrong with me. I think I'm ill. Really irritated that I'm not organized for the day's eating. Had two eggs scrambled with double cream. And had an ounce of cheese.*

Having decaf tea with double cream. Where are the vegetables? This doesn't feel right to me. I just don't feel like I'm on a diet so it makes me nervous.

Feel rubbish and irritated. Had to get out of work today and get some fresh air . . . But I still feel rubbish. Slightly snapped at someone on the phone.

I just don't have a lot of patience today.

I had sliced chicken roast and prawns for lunch with a side salad of spinach.

And have bought a cheap job lot of small water bottles in the hope I'll start drinking more and I'll feel better.

It was my friend's birthday and we did a little party for her at our house in the evening. So much cake and drink going around . . . I had a tiny nibble. Not because I was tempted actually but because I just thought I should join in, but only a tiny nibble. I didn't want to draw attention to myself. Don't think that is the right way to do it though. I have such an all-or-nothing mentality. Need to refresh myself on how to deal with peer pressure. It is amazing to me how being on a diet can make so many people feel they have the licence to comment.

All is fine though. It's nearly 7pm and I'm feeling shattered again . . . and guess what . . . irritated. My poor daughter didn't get a very long bedtime story tonight.

Had some salmon fillets and some veg for supper.

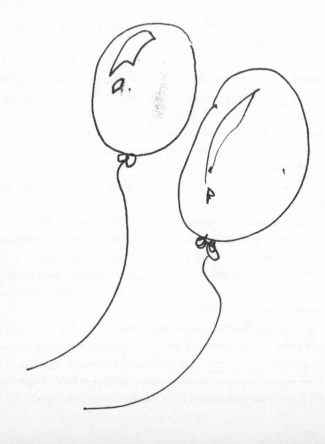

Phase One Day Four

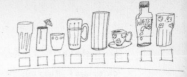

So, Day Four. You may not be feeling that fantastic. You may be wondering if this book comes with a money-back guarantee. Or, you may be thinking, 'My goodness, I have a strange idea that this may be working,' and have a sort of 'thin' feeling, best described as a kind of hollowness. Probably you're somewhere in the middle: you have faith, but, not to put too fine a point on it, you've felt better.

Well, take comfort. It doesn't get much worse than this. Apart from tomorrow. After that, it's plain sailing all the way *provided you don't cheat.* At this stage of the diet, the smallest, titchiest cheat is the kiss of death. It may seem very odd that one little mouthful of toast or a mini-bite of cheesecake should completely derail you and halt your weight loss, but it will. We can't repeat this often enough. Please stick to the programme. You're already losing weight. You have started burning your own fat. Don't stop now. If you have a headache, take paracetamol, and up your water intake. We're sympathetic to your plight, of course. But we also want to make it clear that not feeling 100 per cent is an obstacle that you just have to crash through, which you will, any second now, on your path to slimness. And once you've crashed through it, it's gone for ever.

Besides, if you are feeling rough – Neris felt really grim, India didn't – the thing to bear in mind is that you aren't feeling rough because you've done something terrible to yourself. You're feeling rough because you're detoxing from all the things that are really bad for you, which make you fat, and which will continue to make you fatter and fatter for all eternity unless you get a grip now. Your body is readjusting, that's all. Both it and you will feel much better once the readjustment has occurred. It may help to think of this period as being the equivalent of stopping smoking: a couple of days of mild discomfort in exchange for a lifetime of freedom.

Except that you're not going to fail. Listen, we did it. And we were the least-disciplined, weakest-willed people we know when it came to the question of food. Now, onwards and upwards.

Breakfast

Water and supplements first, remember. Then take your pick from the options on offer, with which you should by now be familiar. Have poached eggs, maybe on a bed of buttered spinach. Or scramble them with a dash of cream, and have some smoked salmon on the side. Or have boiled eggs, perhaps using asparagus spears as soldiers.

But what we would suggest today is that you experiment with breakfast foods which aren't so traditional – like the buttered kippers, the bacon and eggs – and have a go at trying something you would never usually associate with eating first thing in the morning. The truth of the matter is that it is quite possible to get tired of eggs, perfect and speedy as they may be. You can get egged out on this diet if you don't watch out, and so the clever thing to do is never to let yourself get to the 'eggs make me gag' stage.

How do you do this? By having something lunchy for breakfast. Remember: apart from toast and jam, none of the traditional breakfast foods are sweet – not eggs and bacon, not the full English, not salty porridge, not kippers. And yet for some reason many of us have got it into our heads that breakfast must be sugary. I (India) have never had a problem with this – as I was explaining earlier, I prefer salty things to sweet ones, so gorging on pastries, or croissants and apricot jam has never been my bag. I've often had leftovers for breakfast, even before embarking on this way of eating. Personally, I really love left-over curry – sometimes I don't even bother reheating it – but I do see that this might be a bit extreme for most people. But you could ease yourself in the gentler way, perhaps by pretending that you've woken up in Bavaria by accident and therefore have no choice other than to breakfast on cold cuts and cheese. Half of Europe eats this way, so there must be something in it. Ham, smoked meat, salami, cubes of cheese: it's awfully good, and awfully filling. Or try something relatively bland, such as mozzarella dressed with olive oil, torn into pieces and mixed with diced tomato and avocado, and maybe a few basil leaves.

Or have a couple of sticky, caramelized sausages (which you

could have with onion gravy, provided you don't use flour to thicken it). Experiment. You may very well find that last night's roast chicken dipped into a creamy dressing makes a very excellent breakfast indeed.

Useful Tip

There is nothing less satisfying than eating standing up in front of the open fridge door. You may be consuming the right foods, in generous quantities, but you won't feel like you've eaten properly – you'll feel like you've picked at things and had a tiny snack, which means you'll feel grumpy and swizzed. So always, always arrange your food on a large plate. You may think, why bother – I'm in a rush, and I'm only opening a bag of lettuce leaves to go with my Parma ham. But you'd be wrong. Put the ham on the plate. Make a nice little pile of leaves, and dress them. Chop up a tomato. De-stone half an avocado, and anoint it with lime juice and olive oil. Cut yourself a couple of generous chunks of cheese. See? You now have something proper to eat. Even if it's only an assembly job, as opposed to something you've cooked from scratch, eating it served up properly, rather than grabbed on the hoof, can – and does – make all the difference.

Never eat standing up. Never, never, never. Eating standing up makes you dissatisfied. Being dissatisfied makes you eat some more. Ergo, eating standing up makes you fat.

Now, walking. We really hope you've been doing it. It makes a difference, otherwise we wouldn't even suggest it. We were lucky, in that we started our diets in the summer, when walking was relatively pleasant, and usually rain-free. You may not be so lucky: if you're doing this in the depths of winter, the idea of getting off your backside can appear very counter-intuitive.

But you've GOT to do it!

You are going to lose a great deal of weight. To be perfectly honest with you, and very un-PC, you would lose the weight at this stage whether you exercised or not.

BUT: there is no way on earth that you will appear toned if you don't exercise. You will be thin, but floppy.

Later – don't worry: much, much later – we will suggest you step up your exercise a bit if you've lost a great deal of weight, because as we discovered, failure to do so means the formerly fat bits of your body turn into thin but weirdly saggy bits, and this is – obviously – really not at all a good look. But then, we did lose five stone each: it may not be a problem if the shrinkage you have in mind is less drastic.

Still, though, you've got to move around a bit. It speeds up your metabolism, which means you lose weight faster, and walking tones your legs and bottom, which you absolutely need to do if you're planning on losing more than a couple of pounds. If you can bear to do a silly pumping motion with your arms at the same time, it'll work them as well. So get walking. We mean it. Like we keep saying, you're after a degree of breathlessness, but not so much that you huff and puff and go purple in the face.

Walking Dos and Don'ts

Wear proper trainers, even if it means taking your shoes to work in a bag. Not 'fashion' trainers, or the old moth-eaten ones you've had lying around for five years, or the ones that look the most photogenic: wear well-fitting (i.e. snug) ones that won't give you blisters, rub against your toes or flip-flop at the back. And wear socks with them.

Take large strides. You may not be used to them if you live the rest of your life in heels, but tottery little steps aren't what we're after here. Pretend you're wearing seven-league boots.

Comedy arm movements – as if you were a cartoon of somebody walking – it will make you feel slightly embarrassed for the first few days, but then you get used to looking like a fool. They help work the upper body. We suggest you do them.

If you are quite fat, it's entirely likely that your thighs rub together when you walk. Don't use this as an excuse not to do it. Instead, wear thickish trousers rather than a dress (cotton is best – most breathable) and march away, safe in the knowledge that thigh-rub will soon be a thing of the past. If you must walk wearing a dress or skirt, use talcum powder to facilitate slip and minimize rub. Or wear loose men's boxer shorts, which go down past the worst rubby bit. Be prepared for all weather eventualities, so that you don't cut your walk short because it's raining. Buy a lightweight, foldable mac or cagoule (wooh! Lookin' good!) and keep it in your handbag.

Try not to walk carrying something heavy on one side of your body only. If you're carrying shopping bags, spread the weight evenly. If you're lugging heavy things to and from work, buy a backpack. You don't want to knacker your spine. Speaking of which, try and be aware of posture. Often, this means standing up so straight that you feel self-conscious. Do it anyway. Good posture lengthens, and can therefore be quite dramatically slimming. And you'll lose some of the benefits of walking if you do so while sporting the posture of a chimpanzee.

Music can really get you moving: make yourself a walking playlist and download it onto your iPod. All those dancy songs you're slightly embarrassed about still liking – Dead or Alive and Abba, in India's case, Scissor Sisters, Lily Allen and Beyoncé in Neris's. Steer clear of ballads, obviously, or anything that's not frenetically up-tempo. India has tried marching briskly to sonatas, but it doesn't really work. If you have iTunes, there's a ready-made 'Fitness mix' on the iTunes store that you can download, and it's not bad at all.

We swear by MBT, aka Masai Barefoot Technology, trainers. They're not beautiful and they are expensive, but we can't shake off the feeling that they have an extremely effective toning action on the legs, stomach and bottom. See www.mbtshoes.co.uk for information and stockists, but don't get too hung up on this, or think you can't walk properly without them: any well-fitting trainer will do.

Walking with a pram or buggy is great; walking with very little children less so, because they won't be able to keep up with you. You'll both feel miserable about this, so leave them at home. If you're home alone with them, wait until the evening, when you can hopefully park them with someone for a little while. Walking at dusk, or in the dark, can be quite liberating, especially if you feel self-conscious.

Walking with a dog is one of life's great joys.

Walk as fast as you like as your stamina increases over the coming weeks, but don't run. According to a couple of personal trainers we know, almost everybody runs wrongly, in a way that jars their body and impacts badly on their knees – ten years down the line, if not right away. We're not in the business of messing up your joints, or ours, so: don't run. Besides, it can be disastrous on the bust in the long term if you're anything heavier than a B-cup. However, if you absolutely insist on running, either get someone from a gym to show you how to do it properly, or take a look at the Couch (potato) to 5K programme from www.coolrunning.com.

Try to vary your walks. If you're working in the middle of town during the week, then there isn't much you can do about it. But try to find a park or bit of countryside at the weekends – or a beach, if you're lucky enough to live near one. Walking the exact same route every day can get boring (though never mind – the point isn't to thrill you, the point is to make you shrink); walking through a park is much more interesting. Don't be lazy or complacent: if a walk becomes too easy for you, up the tempo. Wear deodorant, and plenty of it. You're going to sweat.

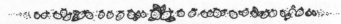

What we have discovered over the course of our time on this diet is this: no matter how grotesquely unfit you are (and India literally hadn't exercised since playing lacrosse, of all absurd things, at school twenty-five years ago), you can become demonstrably fitter in a matter of weeks. This feels utterly fantastic. The downside is, skip exercise for a week or so and your fitness levels plummet in freakishly dramatic fashion. So keep at it.

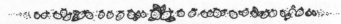

Lunch

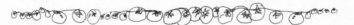

FAUX SHEPHERD'S PIE

FILLING

1.5kg extra lean minced beef
2 medium onions, finely sliced
2 sticks celery, finely chopped
1 tsp fresh thyme leaves
1 tbsp tomato puree
sea salt and black pepper
2 tbsp butter
230g mushrooms, chopped

TOPPING

900g trimmed cauliflower
230g grated cheddar
60ml sour cream
2 tbsp butter
1 egg
8 cooked, crumbled bacon rashers

Put the beef in a large pan and cook over high heat until it stops looking red and raw. Add onions, celery, thyme, tomato puree. Season. Cover, turn heat right down and cook for thirty minutes, stirring from time to time. Add some water if it looks too dry.

Fry the mushrooms in the butter and add to beef; cook for fifteen minutes more.

Meanwhile, make the topping: steam the cauliflower until almost mushy, about fifteen minutes. Blend in food processor, adding cream, cheese and butter. Add the egg and whizz again. Mix in the bacon. Assemble the shepherd's pie and bake at 180°C, gas 4, for forty-five to fifty minutes. Can be made the night before and reheated in the office microwave.

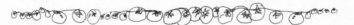

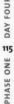

Supper

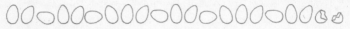

PERFECT ROAST CHICKEN

1 large organic chicken, between 2 and 2.5kg
1 whole onion, peeled
fresh thyme and rosemary, 4 fat sprigs of each OR a handful of fresh
    tarragon
4 garlic cloves, peeled
2 unwaxed lemons
olive oil
sea salt
black pepper

Turn oven on to 190°C, gas 5.

Put the chicken in a roasting tray. Cut the onion into quarters and
shove it inside the cavity. Stick the garlic and herbs in there too (no need
to chop). Cut the lemons in half, squeeze juice over chicken, then cram
the squeezed lemons into the cavity also (quite crowded in there, but
never mind). Anoint the chicken with olive oil – massage it in. Sprinkle
generously with a spoonful or so of sea salt. Season with pepper.

Put chicken in the preheated oven for one and a half hours. Baste
occasionally if you can be bothered – it doesn't make much of a difference
with this method. Let the chicken sit for ten minutes before you carve
it. Use the tin juices as a thin but very flavourful gravy, or add a splash
of double cream for a thicker sauce. Serve with salad, veggies from the
allowed list and/or cauliflower mash. Enough for four.

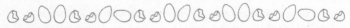

Thought for the Day

You may be disappointed if you fail, but you are doomed,
DOOMED if you don't try.

How We Felt on Day Four

Neris: *Stuck to it pretty much. Weird old day though. Had to go to a funeral three hours away from home. Feeling again . . . guess what . . . Irritated.*

We stopped at a service station in Warwick and had breakfast. Breakfasts are great on this diet. We had egg and bacon and cheese. Lovely. I couldn't drink much water today because we were travelling so much and then at the funeral. So feel a bit sad about that.

The wake was fine. I picked open sandwiches and ate the insides. And had a scoop of double cream that was on the scones. Not a great look but hey it was a funeral and I felt good about doing that. I also had some nuts but I was desperate at that point. Had a dinner of scrambled eggs and loads of cheese.

Upset and irritated and tired. Not a good combination at all.

India: *The thing that is SERIOUSLY getting me down is that I still haven't pooed. For God's sake. Horrible. Gross.*

Headache has increased slightly, but still just about tolerable. Feel quite listless and tired, though. Had long lunch with girlfriend and was pleased to see that there were loads of things I could eat chalked up on the pub blackboard. Had smoked mackerel pâté and soup, and a plate of cheese. I like the fact that I am eating relatively normally, so that there's no need to make a great big song and dance about being on a diet. The one person I've mentioned it to gave me a long lecture about the perils of low-carb diets. Since she's never actually been on one, it all sounded wildly exaggerated. But anyway: apparently her 'friend' who did Atkins had to stop after a couple of days because she kept fainting. Don't understand how you'd possibly faint eating the amounts I've been shoving down. It IS important to remember to eat, though. No skipping meals (as if!).

Evening: headache awful. Achy limbs. Feel slightly fluey. Going to bed early.

Now please read through tomorrow's entry.

Phase One Day Five

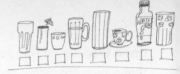

(This may fall on Days Four or Six for some people.)

This was the day we felt *really* bad. On the other hand, some of our guinea-pigs felt absolutely fine – actively great, in a few cases – so here's hoping you do too. See how you feel this morning, and go with it: if you're feeling crap, it may be time to throw a sickie, or call for help with childcare if you're at home with babies. Be absolutely sure to drink your water today, and up the intake a bit if you can bear to – you'll feel better for it. And take things easy: if there's the possibility of spending some time reclining on the sofa in front of the telly, grab it.

Remember, it doesn't get any worse than this. From now on, the only way is up. Also remember – we've said this before, but we'll just say it again – you're not feeling bad because you're doing something terrible to yourself. You're feeling bad because you're detoxing from all the sugar, caffeine and processed rubbish that was clogging up your system and making you fat and unhealthy. Bear with it.

If you're anything like us, today might very well be the day when you have an overwhelming urge to give up. Your mind starts playing funny tricks on you: 'I'm fine as I am,' it tells you. 'So I'm on the podgy side. So what? I'm happy. Life's too short for these kinds of sacrifices. And I want a biscuit.'

It is important that you see this for what it is: a trick. Self-sabotage, to be precise – a talent most serial dieters have in spades. It's time to knock it on the head once and for all. If you were happy with the way you looked, you wouldn't have picked up this book. That's the truth of it. The other truth is that you've nearly completed Week One, and that with this way of eating, as with others, your body is reprogramming itself every day, every hour, every minute. Soon it will barely register irritation (or furious rage) at not having sugary snacks shoved down its gullet every half an hour. So stick with us.

Breakfast

Water and supplements, needless to say, followed by anything
from the allowed list. Or a protein shake, if you don't feel much
like eating. You need one scoop of whey protein powder, which
you get from any health food shop – check the label, please:
some are carbier than others. To your scoop, add a glassful
of *unsweetened* soya milk, and any flavouring you like and are
allowed: vanilla essence (the real thing, not the extract); peanut
butter; a sprinkling of nuts; double cream for added richness.
Whizz it all up (you can do this with a fork – it doesn't go all
lumpy) and drink. This is a useful breakfast if you're in a hurry,
too – it takes ten seconds to make, is protein-packed, and easily
keeps you going until lunch.

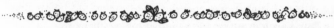

Oh, for God's sake, I really want something sweet! Like, NOW!
Yeah, we know. We personally chose not to go down the artificial
sweetener route, simply because we don't entirely trust them
– we actively despise aspartame (which causes cancer in rats, and
there is, to say the least, a huge question mark over its safety)
and we're not 100 per cent convinced about the safety of the
newer ones, either. But you may feel differently. In that case,
you can have Splenda, which is actually made from sugar (one
carb per sachet). Sweeten the protein shake above with some, or
have sweetened, whipped double cream with a dusting of cocoa
powder and/or nuts. Just don't go making too much of a habit of
it. Sugar got most of us into this mess in the first place. We think
it's better to tell your body that sugar simply no longer features,
but we do realize that this is quite hardcore. Do as you see fit, but
be on your guard. And do try to butch it out for the time being, at
least during Phase One.

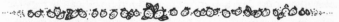

Today is a day when you deserve some cheering up. We hate to venture into women's magazine territory, but sod it, we're going to. The following suggestions may sound like desperate old chestnuts, but we find they work for us. Try not to huff cynically as you read through them. They may very well work for you, too.

Read a book. Go to the bookshop and buy the fattest, trashiest, most engrossing-looking volume you can find. Or buy *The Brothers Karamazov*, by all means, if that's what works for you, or an atlas, or the entire Booker Prize shortlist, or whatever. We like a bit of trash-lit every now and then, ourselves. Make a cup of tea, lie on the sofa, and extract said book from its bag. Not the most original suggestion in the world, granted, but we do guarantee a couple of hours of utter (and distracting) contentment.

Buy some flowers. Flowers make us really happy. Disproportionately so, really, considering that a cheap bunch costs the same as a ready-made cake. Sit and stare at the flowers. Suddenly, life is beautiful. And you're beautiful too. Wussy, but true. Hooray!

Have a hot, fragrant bath. Line the edge of the bath with candles. Put music, or the radio, on. Lie there for hours, until you go all wrinkly. Bliss.

Listen to music. Or tune your radio to BBC 7 and recline, listening to some marvellous old thesp reading stories to you. This works especially well if you're in bed at the time, though your comfiest armchair works well too.

Keep your mind occupied. Obvious, but essential. If you've got nothing to think about other than how not-brilliant you feel, and how you fancy a doughnut, you're actively helping the self-sabotage.

If you can't keep your mind occupied, **do something that requires concentration.** India is a knitting fiend – in fact we'd go as far as saying that, for her, buggering around with wool has been a really marvellous diet aid. Crochet, too – and you can crochet your child (or yourself) a beanie in an evening. Neris paints. Do what you like, even if you haven't done it for years.

Sketching is a heavenly thing to do.

Watch the telly. Rent a DVD, but preferably not *Babette's Feast*.

Lunch

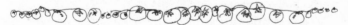

THAI SALMON FISHCAKES

(Serves two as a starter or main, depending on how hungry you are.)

200g salmon
1 red chilli, sliced
4 spring onions
handful fresh coriander, chopped
1 egg
2 teaspoons finely chopped lemongrass (I use 'lazy' lemongrass in jars)
salt and pepper
olive oil

Put everything but the salmon in the blender until finely chopped. Add salmon, salt and pepper to taste, and blend again until similar to mince. It will be quite sloppy, but don't panic!

Heat a good puddle of oil in a frying pan.

Blob tablespoons of the mixture into the pan (makes eight little cakes, or four large ones). If it starts to spit, turn the heat down. Let one side really seal before trying to turn over (like an omelette). When firm and golden brown, they are ready. Delicious served with a squeeze of lime juice and black pepper and stir-fried cabbage.

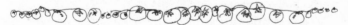

Supper

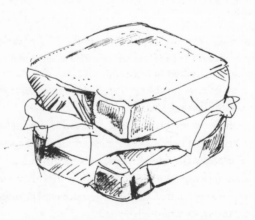

DELICIOUS ASPARAGUS

1 big bundle asparagus
50g unsalted butter
2 hard-boiled eggs
black pepper

Steam the asparagus until done. Meanwhile, gently melt the butter.
Mash the eggs into it, add pepper. Dip the asparagus into the egg-butter
mixture. Total heaven. Serves one greedy person, or two more restrained
types.

How We Felt on Day Five

I think we've covered this. We felt really, really crap. We felt
like Mrs Crappy from Crapville, Crapland, United Crapdom.
Appropriately enough, Day Five was the day India finally
pooed, so there was some rejoicing. But not much.

However . . .

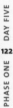

Phase One Day Six

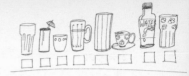

(This may fall on another day for you.)

On Day Six, we felt fabulous. F-A-B-U-L-O-U-S. Fabulous enough for it to be nothing short of miraculous. There we were, dragging ourselves around on Day Five, with the nasty headache and the achy limbs and the weird taste in the mouth and the general 'I'm dying' and 'I can't do it, what's wrong with being fat, anyway?' melodramatic vibe going on, and then, suddenly, on Day Six, we leapt out of bed feeling wonderful and curiously energetic. Hallelujah! And about bloody time, too, frankly.

You may, by the way, experience this first week in a different order from us. You may not have a bad Day Five – you may not have a bad day at all, in which case you can skip this entry. Or you may have more than one, in which case re-read it, for strength. And remember, all the advice and recipes in this section are interchangeable. You don't have to cook the recipes we give you: they're just suggestions. This is a diet book, not a cookbook: cook what you like, sticking to the rules. Just because we don't give a method for crab with spring onions and ginger, or braised belly of pork with star anise, or double-bacon cheeseburgers (sans bun, naturellement, mais avec mayo, gherkins and salsa) doesn't mean you can't eat them. As for the stuff you used to eat: be ingenious about recreating them in a diet-friendly way. Steamed cabbage leaves, for instance, make a nice substitute for lasagne sheets.

But anyway: here we are on Day Six. The sun is shining a little bit more brightly. There's a spring in our step and a song in our heart. For Neris and me, there was also a distinct and unmissable 'thin' feeling. It's hard to put this into words – we just felt lighter, cleaner, better. Whether you are experiencing the thin feeling today, or whether that was yesterday, or whether you've got it to look forward to tomorrow, well done. But be careful. The thin feeling can cause serious wardrobe malfunction. Because it's so pleasing to feel lighter – and tomorrow is weighing day, by the way, so try and resist the temptation to weigh or measure yourself today, no matter how well you feel – the temptation to celebrate the thin feeling sartorially can be overwhelming. I (India) decided on Day Six that I felt so great I should maybe wear a little flouncy above-the-knee dress. Big mistake, because I still weighed fifteen-odd stone. So remember: you will be feeling great, and the chances are that your skin and eyes will have taken a dramatic turn for the better too, but feeling great doesn't mean it's time to slip into the gold lamé hotpants just yet. Bide your time.

Breakfast

Have your supplements, your water and breakfast. Here are some Phase One-friendly 'muffins'.

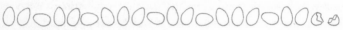

EGG AND SAUSAGE 'MUFFINS'

(makes twelve, which is a lot. Recipe works halved.)

455g sausages
groundnut oil
12 eggs
120ml double cream
120ml water
sea salt
170g grated Cheddar

Preheat the oven to 180°, gas 4. Oil a twelve-cup muffin tray.
Remove the sausages from their skins and fry until browned (with onions if you like; they're nice caramelized). Divide the meat equally between the muffin holes.

Whisk together the eggs, cream, water, salt. Pour over the sausage and top with the cheese. Bake for twenty minutes until golden and fluffy. Cool slightly before attempting to remove from tin.

Feel free to vary this, adding herbs, bacon pieces and so on, and feel free to use any cheese you like.

Now go for your walk.

Today is probably a good day for a little pep talk.

We hope you're discovering for yourself that this diet, or way of eating, is easy to stick to. We hope you're not hungry – if you are, eat more. We hope you've found out that one of the diet's virtues is that it is portable, i.e. that it doesn't ruin your social life; that you can go to restaurants and feast as usual; that cooking at home doesn't involve an unmanageable palaver.

But this is a diet that needs sticking to. You can't (at this stage) go wandering off. You can't think, 'Oh, just this once.' And so today is a good day to ask yourself how you feel vis à vis eating this way in the long term.

Take a good hard look in the mirror (but step off those scales! That's for tomorrow). You should see a distinct improvement. Lie flat in bed and have a feel: there may be some action around your hipbones. Your stomach should be way flatter than it's been for a while. You may even be developing a waist, assuming you thought yours was gone for ever.

Don't stop now. You have achieved all of this in under a week. You are retraining your taste buds, your metabolism, the way your body processes food. You are melting your own fat – and at the rate of knots. You're doing an amazing thing. And if you think you feel good today, just wait another week – and then another month. The results will be jaw-dropping. We promise you.

Don't get complacent. Develop a will of iron. Resist the urge to stick your finger in the Nutella jar. You are going to look fantastic very, very soon. You probably feel pretty great already. Hang on to that feeling, and savour it (as though it were a rose-petal macaroon). You have a choice: either to have that feeling every single day, or to go back to feeling fat, bloated and miserable in changing rooms. The choice is yours, and yours alone.

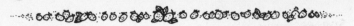

I went to the health food shop this morning and came across an array of low-carb energy bars. Please tell me I can eat them. They're all chocolaty-looking and I feel I deserve a reward!

We wouldn't advise eating them this week or next, i.e. during the stages of Phase One. To be perfectly honest with you, we wouldn't advocate eating them ever – ditto low-carb shakes. The whole point of this diet is to eat 'clean', wholesome food, and to junk the junk, even if the junk ingeniously presents itself as being 'healthy'. The bars you refer to are full of weird stuff – check the ingredients list – and we've yet to find one that tastes anywhere near as good as it looks: nice packaging, but seriously disappointing contents. We also think they can dangerously derail you at this stage – by providing sweetness, which you're trying to teach your body to lose the taste for. They also stall a number of people who follow low-carb, high-protein diets, and the only way to find out you're one of them is to eat them and then watch the scales refuse to budge. But don't panic: another week, and you can have chocolate – real chocolate, not some chemical-laden approximation. We think it's worth waiting for.

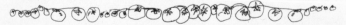

Lunch

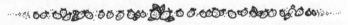

EASY FISH PÂTÉ

Smoked fish
Cream cheese
Juice of 1 lemon
1/2 tsp paprika

Not really a recipe, it's so simple. Also, pleasingly seventies. Get any kind of smoked fish – mackerel, smoked salmon, trout – or any tinned fish you fancy (e.g. tuna). Stick it in the blender with an equal amount of full-fat cream cheese, the juice of a lemon (more if you like it sharper) and half a teaspoon of paprika. Blend. Use crisp lettuce leaves or cucumber sticks to eat off.

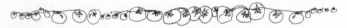

Supper

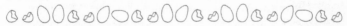

COMFORTING BEEF STEW

1kg lean braising steak
1–2 cloves garlic, sliced or in chunks if you feel brave
A pinch or two of dried chilli
2 large onions
3 courgettes
4–5 field mushrooms
200g broccoli
200g cauliflower
Beef or vegetable stock, approx. 1 pint (depends on size of your
    cooking pot)
2 tbsp olive oil

Chop all veg into big chunks and set aside. Heat the oil in a large
saucepan and brown the meat. Keep frying to seal the meat on all sides
until golden brown. Remove from the pan and set aside on a plate. Fry
the onions and garlic in the pan with the meat juices, allowing to colour
slightly. Return the meat to the pan, adding enough stock to cover. Bring
to a light boil and stir to loosen all the flavour from the bottom. Leave to
simmer gently for one hour with the lid off, until the meat is tender.

Add the veg. You can use any of the vegetables from the 'allowed' list
for this – but remember to put the harder vegetables in first, and the
softer ones last, otherwise they'll turn to mush. Put the lid on and simmer
for a further fifteen to twenty minutes. Serve with a salad and faux-mash
(see page 87 for recipe).

How We Felt on Day Six

Fan-flippin'-tastic!

PHASE ONE   DAY SIX

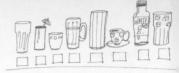

Phase One Day Seven

We would clasp you to our bosoms if we could, and give you a bone-crushing double hug. WELL DONE! You're on the last day of your first week. You have achieved a really wonderful thing. And the hardest bit is over.

We hope you're feeling really, really pleased with yourself. If you're anything like us, you'll be practically mad with joy. We repeat: well done, hooray, hats off and bravo. If this book were interactive, we'd pause for a little triumphant trumpet tune.

Breakfast

Have your supplements, your water and your breakfast.
We suggest sausages. Perfect Fried Sausages.

Here's how to cook them (no, we haven't gone mad, giving you a sausage recipe. It's just that a lot of people don't cook them for long enough, with the result that they taste unpleasantly pink 'n' porky. There's nothing worse than a sausage that's rare in the middle, plus it can make you mighty sick).

So: your frying pan. A nut of butter, a dot of groundnut oil. Get it nice and hot. Add the sausages. Now turn the heat down to the minimum and leave them alone for at least twenty minutes. Then turn them over and repeat on the other side. The result is a really regal sausage, sticky and caramelized on the outside and cooked properly within. While they're cooking, if you can be bothered, very finely slice some onions, fry them on a very gentle heat in some butter (with our friend the dot of oil to avoid burning) until they've gone brown at the edges; toss in some herbs (thyme is nice) and a little liquid – leftover stock, leftover gravy, a corner of stock cube, or even just water, and simmer the whole thing until it's all melted and melded together. Eat with the sausages. Very, very nice. But failing the onion marmalade, try dipping your sausages in any creamy dressing you like, in shop-brought salsa, or in mustard thinned down with sour cream, to which you might add snipped chives.

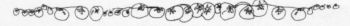

As you are no doubt aware, today is weighing day. 'O frabjous day! Callooh! Callay!' Less poetically, please make sure you've pooed before you step on the scales.

And away you go. Go on, step on them. You have nothing to fear. If you have been following our instructions, you'll have dropped a load of weight. And, by the way, it's not all water-weight – that only happens for the first few days. You've dropped a combination of water-weight and FAT. Congratulations.

Weighing's not enough. Get out the tape measure, too, and measure the parts of your body we mentioned on page 72. Nice, innit? We told you it worked.

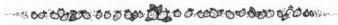

If you haven't lost any weight, you haven't been following the diet properly. It's as simple as that. You've either cheated, or some carbs have snuck in when you weren't looking – your sausages, for example, may have contained bread or other carby fillers; you might have eaten your fish battered without thinking; that jar of shop-bought sauce may have contained starch and sugars. Vigilance, my dears, at all times. We mean it when we say, as we have been over the past week, that the smallest indulgence will completely derail the diet at this stage. Consider yourself chastised and go back to Day One. And don't feel too sad: just put it down to experience. It's not going to happen again. The thing about our diet is, it works. All you have to do is do it properly.

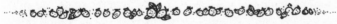

The rest of you will be feeling jubilant. As you should be. And it's only Day Seven. Just wait. Your process of transformation has only just begun.

Now go for your walk, skippety-skipping with joy. Why not add on an extra five or ten minutes? The diet's working, you're already looking and feeling better: go on. You have nothing to lose but your flab.

By the way, just because you've lost weight DOES NOT mean that you can take it easy in terms of food today. No sneaky rewards, please. Have a salon-quality facial instead. Here are some tips, courtesy of celebrity uber-facialist Amanda Lacey:

Home Facials
A Step-by-Step Guide

It is always best to perform your pampering facial last thing in a busy day. Put aside twenty to thirty minutes and remember, when it comes to massage, this should be for at least ten minutes at a time.

Fill a very clean bathroom basin with hot water and throw in a couple of pure cotton-towelling face mitts.

Use a natural oil-based cleanser so as not to dry out the skin too much – we like Amanda Lacey's own cleansing pomade, Eve Lom's eponymous cleanser, or Vaishaly Patel's wonderful cleansing balm, but we're a bit deluxe about cleansers – your local chemist will stock plenty of cheaper alternatives. These waxy cleansers will have a far more effective action on the skin than cream or frothy cleansers, plus they keep skin soft and supple, not stripped and tight feeling. Do not fear them if your skin is oily – it may sound counter-intuitive to use an oily-feeling, waxy product on oily-feeling skin, but trust us, it works.

Warm the cleanser between the palms and massage onto dry skin using upward circular movements.

Grab your mitts and gently exfoliate in small circular motions to remove any dead skin cells from the epidermis (top layer of the skin). This will revive sluggish, sallow complexions and brighten the skin.

Wash your face in a new basin of warm water and make sure every trace of cleanser has been removed.

Pat dry and leave your face alone for one minute. Then sit down and hold your face gently in the palms of your hands. The reason for doing this is that you have just stripped the skin of its pH balance of 5.5. By holding your face you are keeping it warm and therefore retaining the moisture and preventing it from feeling tight (this is especially important in winter months).

Take a drop of facial oil – any kind: most cosmetics companies do one – and warm it between your palms. Then begin to massage it into the skin. If you have time, try to lie on your bed as this will relax you and your facial muscles. Tissue off any excess oil, though there shouldn't be any. At this point you can either go straight to bed or . . .

If you have extra time, you can use a hydrating mask to nourish and soothe dry or irritable skin. The best thing to do is wrap your hair up, put the mask on and soak in a hot bath, removing the mask before you go to bed and finishing off with another drop of face oil.

Amanda's products can be bought from www.amandalacey. com, Vaishaly Patel's from www.vaishaly.com, and Eve Lom's from www.evelom.com. We also recommend Liz Earle's products, available from www.lizearle.com.

Lunch

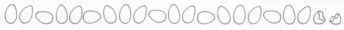

INDIAN SCRAMBLED EGGS

2 eggs
small handful chopped coriander
1 small onion, very thinly sliced
1 green chilli (less if you fear heat)
1 tomato
pinch ground cumin
pinch ground coriander
butter
drop of groundnut oil
salt and pepper

Melt the butter with a drop of oil. The smaller the pan, the less contact with direct heat, and the fluffier the eggs will be. When hot, add onion slices and fry until coloured and crispy around the edges. Meanwhile, mix all remaining ingredients. Tip into the pan containing the onions and scramble for a couple of minutes, or until set. This makes a fantastic brunch dish. Makes one generous portion.

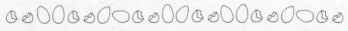

Supper

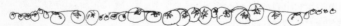

MARINATED SPICED LAMB

2 French-trimmed racks of lamb
3 garlic cloves, crushed
2 tsp ginger, grated
2 tsp white wine vinegar
handful finely chopped mint leaves
2 tsp ground cumin
2 tsp ground coriander
1 tsp chilli powder
150ml yogurt
sea salt

Put the lamb in a shallow dish. Blend together the garlic, ginger, vinegar, mint, cumin, coriander, chilli, salt and yogurt in a food processor. Pour this mixture over the lamb, cover, and refrigerate for at least three hours (overnight is best).

When ready to eat, preheat the oven to 200°C, gas 6. Lay the lamb on a lined baking sheet and cook for twenty minutes if you like it pink, longer if you don't. Remove from oven and allow to rest for ten minutes before cutting into cutlets. Serves four.

How We Felt on Day Seven

Happy, happy, happy.

Phase One Day Eight

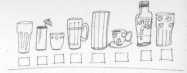

Look at the time, already. You're on the first day of your second week. No mean feat, you know.

Basically, what happens now is that we carry on as we were. Week Two is a repeat of Week One. You've presumably got the gist by now. Keep sticking to the rules, keep drinking your water and taking your supplements, and keep walking. Remember, if it starts feeling too easy, up the tempo and add on five minutes.

We're not going to give you any more recipes for this second week. Repeat those for Week One, if you're not tired of them, and if you are, use your existing cookbooks, or improvise.

Here are some breakfast ideas:

- Eggs and bacon
- Vegetable omelettes
- Cheese and ham omelettes
- Scrambled eggs with crab
- Pigs in blankets
- Poached eggs on spinach, with hollandaise sauce
- Poached eggs on ham, with hollandaise sauce
- Frittatas
- Creamed mushrooms
- Grilled tomatoes
- Avocados – sliced into an omelette if you prefer
- Buttered kippers
- A cup of vegetable soup, with added olive oil and/or parmesan, and added crunchy bits of bacon, if you like
- A cup of instant miso soup
- A handful of nuts
- Leftover roast meats with dressing
- The antipasti option – hams, salamis, cheeses, olives

Anything at all, really, from your list of allowed foods. As we've been saying, there is no law that decrees that breakfast must be bready, or sugary, or grainy. You want prawns dipped into mayo for breakfast? Go right ahead. It's not as odd as it sounds, as you're hopefully discovering by now.

And if you're in a rush, remember the protein shake recipe on page 119.

Time to look, now, at swapping bad habits for good. We've established that you'll soon be able to have some fruit, porridge for breakfast (or whenever you prefer) and even the odd chunk of chocolate. All of that happens next week. In the meantime, here's what to do when you crave a particular thing.

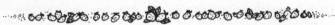

FRUIT! I want fruit! And fruit is good for you, so why can't I have it?

The truth of the matter is that fruit is only good for you up to a point. Vegetables are much better. This is because fruits contain sugar, as fructose, and we're trying to steer clear of sugars for the time being – which means steering clear of anything that ends in '-ose', including fructose. Citrus fruits – the breakfast orange juice which we believed for so long was incredibly good for us – are now avoided by many people and by many complementary therapists, not least because they're awfully acidic, especially on an empty stomach: hello, reflux. Bananas are yummy, but they're the fruit equivalent of the potato: carb city. From next week, you'll be allowed berries and melons, so don't get your knickers in a twist and just bear with us. In time, when you've lost the bulk of your weight, you'll be able to have any fruit you like, though we'll encourage you to choose your fruit with care and not to go guzzling vast quantities willy-nilly.

PORRIDGE! I want porridge! And porridge is good for you too, so why can't I have that either?

It is good for you, yes – and it keeps you going, as well. But it's still too carby for Phase One. However, you can have it regularly from Phase Two onwards, so hang in there.

I want a pudding.

Do you really, though? It's Day Eight and you've done brilliantly so far. But if you must, then have whipped double cream sweetened with Splenda, to which you can add chopped nuts and vanilla essence. Have this in a normal-sized bowl please, not a trough. From today you're also allowed sugar-free jelly, with whipped cream (but NOT the stuff out of a can).

I want something crunchy, like crisps or biscuits.

Make Parmesan wafers. Coarsely grate Parmesan, or cheddar, or a mixture of the two. Add cayenne if you like a bit of heat with your crunch. Cover a baking sheet with baking parchment or those clever silicone non-stick sheets (good investment, plus they last for ever). Pile on the cheese in little clusters – space them far apart, because obviously they're going to melt. Stick them in a preheated oven (190°C, gas 5) and watch them like a hawk – they only take a few minutes. Cool them (this is crucial). Peel them off. If they've all melted into one big sheet, break it apart. And lo: we have crunch. Keep in an airtight box, if they last that long – they're very moreish.

You can also have nuts, for crunch. And very crispy bacon rashers. And, should it be your bag, pork scratchings.

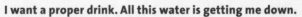

I want a proper drink. All this water is getting me down.
And you shall have one next week – it'll be double voddies all round. Clean spirits contain no carbs, but we're taking them out of Phase One because we didn't find it helpful to drink while we were at this stage of the diet. Spirits may be carb-free, but when there is alcohol present in your system, your body will burn it for fuel first, i.e. while it's doing this, it won't be burning your own fat. Also, there is always the danger of having one drink too many and thinking, 'Ah, sod it, I want a bag of chips' and acting on that slightly drunken impulse. Which would be disastrous at this stage.

So for the moment, please stick to the water and tea or coffee. The water is your friend. The water is helping you get thin.

Remember, you can use soya milk to create your own version of a latte. And here's how to make a homemade chai latte: put a big mugful of soya milk in a saucepan. Add two crushed cardamom pods, half a stick of cinnamon, a clove, a slice of fresh peeled ginger, two teabags (or two scoops of tea-leaves) and a pinchlet of Splenda. Heat until just before boiling point. Strain. Heaven.

I feel like I'm eating industrial quantities of meat. I know I'm a carnivore, but this is ridiculous.
Well, then eat less of it. India ate a lot of seafood but not much fish before embarking on this diet – something to do with being nervous about cooking it. No more. Fish rocks, it's easy to cook, and it takes hardly any time to prepare. Do not fear it. And do not fear tofu, either.

I want chocolate.

Us too. The point here is that it's not only your body or taste buds that we need to re-educate. It's also your mind that needs reprogramming. We bumble along through life thinking, 'This is just the way I am,' or, 'This is just the way I think,' so that when our mind says, 'Time for biscuits,' we just think, 'Oh, okay,' and mindlessly reach for the cookie jar. It's all well and good, thinking this is just how we are – but when it comes to food, it's also not true.

Eating two Danish pastries for breakfast is not the way you are meant to live at all. It's not the way you were born. It has very little to do with anything, except habit. And all habits are breakable. If people can get off heroin, you can get off thinking that you're doing yourself a favour by eating fattening crap. Be the boss of yourself, as my children would say. When you have the thought that says, 'Bugger it, I want to eat the garlic bread,' don't just give in to it spinelessly. Hold it up for examination (the thought, not the bread) instead of frantically trying to push it aside. Have a good look at it, and then dismiss it. Don't try to push the thought away halfway through having it, or get in a panic about it – that's how obsessions are created, and how you end up feeling deprived instead of in control.

Hold it in your head and examine it. All you have to tell yourself is, 'Actually, that's a crap idea. I'm getting thinner. Why would I have the garlic bread? I'd be mad to.' If you do this enough – and admittedly it is quite boring, but also important – it becomes second nature. What we're basically saying is, never take any food-related thought you have for granted. Ever. Examine it. Show it who's boss: you, and you alone.

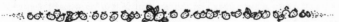

Some More Ideas for Lunch

The antipasto plate, but this time including a couple of semi-dried tomatoes (delicious: they taste almost candied), artichoke hearts, bottled peppers in olive oil, some more olives, and a big side salad, with cheese if you like.

Any salad – but be butch about it, and not namby-pamby. Salads don't have to be wimpy rabbit food. Add grilled chicken, poached eggs, crispy bacon, hunks of cheese, our old friend the avocado – whatever takes your fancy from the allowed list. A little gem salad with roast chicken and lots of fresh tarragon leaves in a creamy dressing is a very delicious thing indeed. As is a Caesar salad without the croutons. And you're allowed pesto, so either drizzle it on fish or chicken, or use it as a salad dressing.

Vegetable soup, to which you add extra virgin olive oil and Parmesan – and bacon or pancetta, if you like. This is a very useful thing to make a big pot of twice a week, because then you barely have to think. Plus, it freezes beautifully and reheats in minutes. Chicken soup is also very useful, and marvellously comforting.

If you are fortunate enough to live near a fishmonger's, a dressed crab or six oysters make a really wonderful and luxurious treat – and there's no preparation required. Also, those jars of French fish soup are pretty delish (if sometimes a bit salty), especially if you have them with grated Gruyère.

Those low-effort lunch ingredients from the deli aisle are also very useful: don't discount them because they're more traditionally eaten with bread. Have the chicken liver pâté, or the smoked mackerel; the smoked salmon or trout or eel; the soft cheeses. Either train yourself to eat them as they are, or use celery or another robust green vegetable, such as green beans, to scoop.

Guacamole (chop up avocado, tomato, coriander, onion, chilli, squirt with lime juice), see above for dipping materials. Also quite nice scooped out of the bowl with your finger, actually.

A big pot of chilli con carne is a very useful thing to have lurking around in your fridge. Don't include the kidney beans at this stage – but do decorate your portion(s) of chilli with sour cream and chopped avocado if you fancy them.

Supper

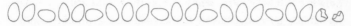

GRILLED PORTOBELLO MUSHROOMS WITH BLUE CHEESE DRESSING
(serves four)

100 g Gorgonzola or other blue cheese, crumbled
4 tbsp sour cream
1 tbsp mayonnaise
1 tbsp red wine vinegar
1 tsp minced garlic
4 portobello mushrooms
extra virgin olive oil
salt and pepper

Mash the cheese to a paste. Stir in the sour cream, mayonnaise, vinegar and garlic. Season to taste.

Remove the stem from each mushroom and scrape out the gills with a small spoon. Score the tops in a cross-hatch pattern. Season the mushrooms with the olive oil, salt and pepper. Grill, two to three minutes on each side until cooked through. Drizzle the dressing on top.

Serve with a green salad.

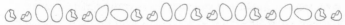

How We Felt on Day Eight
Optimistic.

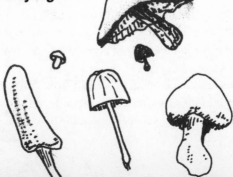

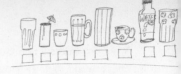

Phase One Day Nine

We're really rolling now.

Eat breakfast. Take your supplements. Drink your water. Go walkies.

Being Prepared, and Why It Really Matters

We can't emphasize this enough: preparation is all. This diet is incredibly easy to follow if your fridge is ready for it, and not so easy if it isn't. If you work long hours, or live miles away from the shops, your new way of eating is going to require forward planning. You do get hungry on this way of eating, and if there's nothing suitable to hand, you're likely to grab the wrong thing, simply because your body is telling you to eat. And that's a big fat disaster.

Unfortunately, the kind of food you're eating is the opposite of the kind of stuff you can keep in the cupboard – no rice, no pasta, no other useful starches or grains. Pretty much everything you're eating is made from scratch and involves fresh ingredients. It may sound like advice from the Good Housekeeping Institute in the 1950s, but with this diet, it really, really pays to sit down on a Friday evening and plan your meals for the following week. That way, your time spent at the shops on Saturday will be intelligently spent. The alternative, if you're me (India), is to do a mad, hurried dash round the supermarket and end up with far too much food, bought on the basis that it's bound to come in handy and it's allowed.

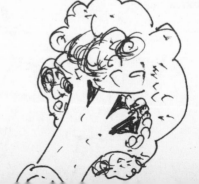

We don't know what your own personal tastes are, obviously, but here is a sample shopping list that should last you a good few days. We like this shopping list. If anyone tells you that the way you're eating is unhealthy, show it to them. We bet it's a great deal healthier than theirs.

- Organic eggs
- Rooibos tea, or herbal tea of your choice
- Two cartons unsweetened organic soya milk
- Butter
- Large carton double cream
- Bacon, smoked or green, preferably cured without nitrates
- Ham, any kind, preferably cured without sugar
- Salami, chorizo, quails' eggs to snack on (with celery salt)
- Walnuts, pine nuts, almonds to snack on
- A hunk of Parmesan
- A hunk of cheddar
- Mozzarella
- One organic chicken
- Another meat of your choice – anything from minced beef to veal cuts for osso bucco
- Fresh fish or seafood (but eat it the day of purchase)
- Firm tofu
- Fresh spinach
- Fresh mushrooms
- Fresh tomatoes
- Fresh salad, and salad vegetables, including chives, cucumber, radishes
- Fresh avocados
- Fresh cauliflower
- Fresh broccoli
- Any extra seasonal green leafy vegetables you fancy
- Fresh herbs of your choice
- Onions
- Garlic
- Olives

- Good olive oil
- Groundnut oil
- Mayonnaise, if you don't make your own
- Sour cream
- Canned tuna (you'll never starve if you have canned tuna to hand)
- Canned tomatoes (but watch out for added sugar)
- Splenda, if you use it
- Whey protein powder
- Vanilla extract

Now here's what a non-dieter might purchase instead:
- Battery eggs
- Normal tea or coffee
- Cow's milk or artificial creamer
- Margarine or 'fake' butter spread
- Large carton ice cream
- Crisps to snack on
- Biscuits to snack on
- Chocolate to snack on
- Processed cheese
- Battery chicken
- Mechanically recovered 'meat' products
- Fish fingers or frozen battered fish
- Frozen peas and another vegetable or two if you're lucky
- Canned fruit in syrup
- Canned soup
- Sugar
- Cakes
- Bread

QED. Anyone who tells you this diet isn't healthy – because they believed all the scare stories about Atkins and eating mince fried in lard three times a day – has not got the full picture. And remember: good plans shape good decisions. The contents of your fridge are the foundation of this diet.

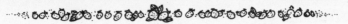

I buy ready meals a lot. I live alone and they're just really convenient. You're going to tell me to give them up, aren't you?
Not necessarily. But you are going to have to turn into Miss Marple and scrutinize the packaging with enormous care. The majority of ready meals use starches as fillers, and they're usually full of flour and sugar, as well – to say nothing of really bad trans-fats. Obviously, this won't do.

However, they're not healthy, and so it's no great loss. On the other hand, they are massively convenient. We suggest you eat better ones less often. The most expensive ones (they would be, wouldn't they?) are the ones formulated with the least additives and the fewest chemicals and E numbers. We particularly like Marks & Spencer's Cook! range. At the time of writing, about seventy per cent of its products are suitable.

I do a weekly supermarket trawl for things like water and loo paper, but then I rely quite heavily on the corner shop. Is there anything at all I can eat that's quick to make and buyable from my local convenience store?
To be honest, your options are going to be really limited – also, it's a really expensive way of shopping. You can buy the ingredients for an omelette, or a cheese plate (maybe), or for a big tuna salad, but beyond that things are probably going to get a bit repetitive. If you like shopping daily broaden your net and find a street with a good grocer and a decent butcher or fishmonger. Then it becomes simple: a piece of grilled chicken, some roast pumpkin to go with it, and a salad on the side. Easy.

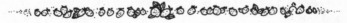

Useful Tip

If you physically go to the supermarket rather than ordering online, avoid the biscuit, cake and crisp aisles for the first few weeks of this eating plan. There's no point at all in putting yourself in temptation's way. Sooner rather than later, these aisles will hold no fear for you. We now blithely skip about every aisle of the supermarket, and buy 'forbidden' foods for our families without batting an eyelid.

Needless to say, it is a really, really bad idea to go food shopping on an empty stomach. Don't make life difficult for yourself: eat first. If you've forgotten, head for the nut aisle, grab some shelled pistachios, or whatever nut you like best, and eat them before you carry on. Remember to hold on to the empty packet, as you still have to pay for them!

Here are some more basic takeaway-style lunch and dinner ideas:

Almost any Indian curry, served with pickles but without rice or bread: chicken tikka masala, for instance, with a side of fragrant spiced spinach and another of cauliflower bhaji

- Thai green or red curry
- Clear Thai soups/broths, such as Tom Yum
- Satay
- Stir fries
- Chicken with cashew nuts
- Chinese-style spare ribs
- Lemon chicken
- Chicken or prawns or fish or crab with spring onions and ginger
- Beef or chicken or pork in satay sauce
- Tiger prawns
- Wok-fried scallops
- Bok choi, or any Chinese greens, either with garlic or with oyster sauce

As you can see, eating this way is not difficult if you're after something yummy to scoff in front of the telly. Having said that, though, try not to scoff in front of the telly. You end up eating in a completely absent-minded and repetitive way, which means that you usually end up eating far more than you needed to. Eat at the table, like a normal person.

How We Felt on Day Nine

India: *I used to do a funny thing when I was really fat: I was incapable of eating by myself, just looking at my plate. I had to have distraction, in the form of either a book or magazine, or the telly. It was as though I knew that physically seeing the amount of stuff I was proposing to wolf down would probably freak me out a bit. Stands to reason, really – I was in denial about what I was eating. So I shovelled it in without actually properly looking at it, staring at a magazine instead. Weird, isn't it? This is one of the many reasons why we would really encourage you to eat sitting at a properly laid table, with a napkin, with cutlery, with a jug of water, whether you are eating alone or with somebody else. You need to focus on what you are doing, and that can't be done with distractions other than conversation. It also means that you'll know when you feel full, rather than just mindlessly carrying on chomping long after you might have stopped.*

Neris: *I felt okay.*

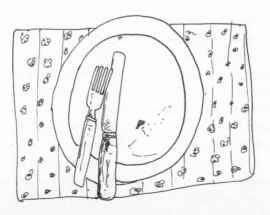

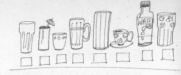

Good morning. We hope it's getting easier, that your clothes are getting looser, and that you're feeling better than you have done in years.

Drink your water. Take your supplements. Eat your breakfast. Walk. If you haven't upped your walking time by at least ten minutes over the past week or so, do it now. If you're marching away for half an hour or more, well done. You'll get to goal (aargh! what a phrase) much faster.

This chapter is especially for you if you have children. As we were saying much earlier on in the book, having young children in particular is often the beginning of the end as far as your waistline is concerned: somehow, mothers feel duty-bound to hoover up their children's leftovers – even if they don't normally particularly like apple purée or fish fingers and chips. Maybe it's some strange biological imperative. And when you add those leftovers to the three adult meals a day you're also eating – well, it's a wonder every fertile woman in the country isn't Zeppelin-shaped.

Obviously, you haven't – we most sincerely hope – been hoovering up those cold, congealed titbits for the past nine days. But here are a few coping strategies to see you through the coming weeks.

First of all, always, always have a snack – or your meal – before you start cooking for children. You're unlikely to lust after their leftovers if you're feeling stuffed.

Secondly, ask yourself if your children really need to eat that differently from you. The truth of the matter is that, Jamie Oliver notwithstanding, we still feed our children an awful lot of junk – we know it's not especially good for them, but every once in a while, we feel we're giving them a treat. But if you cook home-made burgers rather than frozen ones, you know exactly what's gone into them, and you can eat them too. If you swap fish fingers for, say, lemon sole strips pan-fried in butter, you can hoover up all the leftovers you like. If they're having fresh vegetables rather than oven chips, you're more than welcome to help yourself. It makes it all so much easier – and you are dramatically improving your children's health in the process. Leave them to chomp on their bread, potatoes, pasta and rice – they're growing children, and it's not doing them any harm, although if you are seriously concerned about optimizing their physical well-being, swap anything they eat that's white for the brown equivalent – that way, you'll soon be able to join in with those bits, too. So: wholemeal bread, stone-ground; brown or wild rice; and whole foods instead of processed.

If you persuade them to eat this way now – and nothing is more persuasive than leading by example – they'll not only grow up having a healthy idea of what eating well means, but they'll be in peak form physically. And hopefully the patterns that turn us all into fat adults won't ever be in place. Especially if you ensure they cut down on the sugar.

There isn't a recipe in this book that our children would be unhappy to eat, but obviously it's all subjective. Develop your own repertoire of family-friendly recipes that you can all eat together. That way, you don't feel like you're sitting there in miserable, self-imposed exile – you eat what they're eating, but without the stodge.

Eating out with children needn't be tricky either. If the pizza restaurant you're in won't run to a salad, you can eat the pizza topping provided you leave the crust (we don't recommend you do this every day, but once every now and then won't hurt). It doesn't look especially charming, but it's not going to ruin your diet. If you're at a burger joint, tuck in, but leave the bun (and the ketchup, which is mostly sugar). Fried chicken isn't recommended, but provided you pick away the batter, it's not going to harm you – ditto battered fish. Like we keep saying, this is a sociable diet. You're never going to starve – not unless you're locked in a sweet shop or a potato-processing plant.

Back at home, there is an ultra simple solution to not being tempted by the children's crisps, biscuits and cakes: don't buy them. They can have them at friends' houses, but it won't kill them not to have them at home.

Having said that, everybody's different, but we found we didn't have to go to these lengths: once the weight begins to fall off – as you are experiencing right now – the temptation to cock it all up for a mouthful of something sugary fades.

How We Felt on Day Ten

Like we were getting there.

India: *Day Twenty* [India may have been further along in the diet than you are, but we hope this will prove to you that it is possible to feed your kids those forbidden foods without giving into temptation yourself.]

Baked a cake! How perverse is that. Didn't even lick the spoon clean of batter. Have developed a sort of revulsion towards doughy things. Don't know if this is because I have been reading so many low-carb texts and books, but now I just see them as empty and puffy and fatty and bleh. Must watch out for this – don't want to develop a weird nutty obsession about the evils of carbs.

We actually bought exactly what we'd usually buy for our children. This is a way of eating that's life-long, and we felt that the sooner we got used to it, the better. Part of getting used to it means ignoring the three kinds of cereal sitting on top of the fridge. Anyway, we don't really believe that the cereals, or the biscuits, constitute 'temptation'. The idea that some foods are more 'tempting' than others is another clever trick by the diet industry. We believe that everything is about choice: about choosing to make a difference to the way you look by choosing to eat a certain way. If you feel like you're the one wielding the power – which you are – then no amount of sugary carbs will deter you from your chosen path, because the choice is stark and simple: follow the diet, and you lose weight and look great. Ignore the diet because you feel 'tempted', and you get fatter and look worse. It's a no-brainer.

Phase One Day Eleven

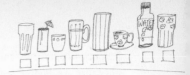

Take your supplements. Drink your water. Have breakfast.
Go for your walk.

By Day Eleven India was in the swing of things; Neris had
a down day and was majorly fed up. Chances are that you may
be too. This diet is easy, and this diet works, but that doesn't
mean that, in its early stages, it can't feel repetitive and slightly
monotonous. We wouldn't blame you if, by today, you're
beginning to think, 'That's enough of that.'

Neither would we blame you if you were thinking, 'This
is great – I could go on for ever.' But for the purposes of this
chapter, we're going to assume that you may be struggling.

It's more an emotional struggle than a physical one – after all,
you're eating, your body is functioning, and you're losing weight.
You should also have noticed a marked improvement in your
energy levels: all that feeling tired at around 4pm is on the way
out. And all of this is good. But one of the really boring things
about diets in the long term is that the pounds only come off as a
result of you making thousands of right decisions, and sometimes
hundreds of the wrong ones. And all of the onus is on you: you're
the only one there for every single one of those choices/decisions.
It can feel quite lonely, or quite overwhelming, or emotionally
exhausting.

Neris: *I always feel a bit short changed when I've got to the end of
a really successful day and just managed to stay on track. What I
remember is all the opportunities that I've turned down. The slice of
birthday cake. The crisps in the bar. The drink at the leaving do. So
many times I could have slipped up – and I didn't. But you don't really
get praised for that. And sometimes you feel like a pat on the head.*

First, consider your head patted. Secondly, we share your
pain. Getting through a day when there are more obstacles to
surmount than usual can feel like you've climbed Everest, except
that instead of there being a celebratory party waiting for you at

the summit, nobody's noticed. And that can make you feel quite resentful. And when you feel resentful, if you're anything like us, the temptation is to reach for your comforting little friend, food.

We'd expect your weight loss by now to be visible. Not dramatically so – nobody's going to come running up to you and exclaim, 'Oh my goodness, how much have you lost?' But it should certainly be visible to you. As far as other people are concerned, you may be getting a number of those 'You look well, what have you done?' comments. Enjoy them. In another fortnight, there will be a physical difference in you that you'd have to be blind to ignore – especially if you have a great deal of weight to lose. This is the image that you have to hold in your head when you're feeling wobbly. Weight loss is no longer an unattainable ideal: you're experiencing it right now. It's no longer pie in the sky. Your clothes should be feeling looser already, and pretty soon you're going to have to chuck them away because they'll be ridiculously big on you. That's not wishful thinking; it is fact. You've got to hang on in there.

If you're feeling that the diet is monotonous, take heart from knowing that you only have another three days to go before it broadens out a great deal and allows you, among other things, alcohol and chocolate. Three days out of your whole life is not a high price to pay for being the shape you want to be.

While Neris was feeling irritated on Day Eleven, I knew I'd cracked it. The point of telling you this isn't that I was a good girl and that she was naughty. It is that we both got there in the end, following different routes. You're allowed to have wobbles, to feel annoyed or restricted or both, just as (obviously) you're allowed to find this way of eating pretty effortless and simple. Whether you're finding things easy or hard doesn't really matter when it comes to the end result, because provided you don't waver, you will lose all the weight you want to lose. Sure, there's an easy way to do this – which is just to do it, without questioning anything. And there's a harder way – which I expect occurs when people (Neris being a prime example) are dieters of many years' standing. The harder way involves feeling deprived and querying everything you aren't allowed to put in your mouth – 'But WHY can't I have a cup of hot chocolate?' Well, you know the answer to that one, so my advice would be, don't even go there. You might as well ask, 'But WHY can't I inject my eyeballs with heroin?' You could, you know. You are a free agent – if that's what you really want, go ahead. But you'll have failed to look after yourself, and you'll have cocked up. You'll also be setting a dangerous precedent. And if you cock up, you have to start all over again.

Okay. You know what? I'm happy to start all over again, provided you allow me to cock up today. You said I could go off-piste in the introduction, after all.

We simply can't emphasize this enough: at this stage of the diet, going off-piste is fatal. Your body is getting used to this new way of eating, and getting into the swing of burning your own fat as fuel. If you give it extra carbohydrates to use as fuel instead, it'll go off the rails. It is entirely possible that you will put on up to five pounds overnight, or within twenty-four hours. Seriously. We really, really advise you not to go there – because on top of everything else, those extra pounds won't just fall off when you get back on the diet; they'll hang around for a while and may prove hard to shift.

Phase Two of the diet allows you to fall off the wagon occasionally. Phase One doesn't. So don't. If you already have, and are reading this too late, go back to Day One and start all over again. Here's another thing you should know about the diet: it works brilliantly the first time. And it works okay the second time. By the third time, your metabolism doesn't quite know what to do with itself; everything slows down dramatically, and the diet only half works. Alarming, but true – it's true of every diet. Let's not even go into the fourth or fifth time: it'll still work eventually, but we're talking months and months rather than weeks. Don't mess it all up for the sake of a Twix.

I don't know what you're talking about in this chapter. I feel really inspired.

We're delighted to hear it. I (India) felt really inspired too, especially when I noticed a difference in the way my clothes fitted around the waist. After horrible Day Five was over, and to this day, I like everything about this diet. I like how it's easy and I don't have to think – only occasionally read labels carefully; I like how it's easy to incorporate into my social life; I like – love – the way it makes me feel; and above all, I like the fact that it works. I've always liked cooking, and I like ploughing through my recipe books to find more and more things to cook. I have to say, liking cooking – which Neris doesn't, particularly – has made this way of eating 100 per cent easier: I really enjoy the fact that I can go through my favourite books and find literally hundreds of recipes that work just as they are, and which don't even need adapting. So if you're feeling inspired, good on you. Carry on. You have a huge advantage over the people who are struggling a bit. But you'll both get there in the end.

So what did Neris do? Deep breath . . .

So you're well into the second week. Hopefully you've thought about why you got fat in the first place, learnt the rules of what to eat, and started the actual diet. But now comes the tricky bit – sticking to it. I failed many times before I succeeded, always promising myself that 'this time it's going to be different'. So what has changed?

Here is my diary entry from thirteen months ago:

I can't do this. I don't know what's wrong with me. Oprah Winfrey's epiphany came when she was standing on the verandah of her new-colonial mansion in Hawaii, celebrating her fiftieth birthday. She looked at everything she had achieved, and how far she had come, and finally it clicked. However rich she was, she would never be truly happy while she was overweight.

I wanted my epiphany, when everything would suddenly make sense. I was overweight and unhappy as well. I didn't even have the mansion in Hawaii. To be honest, my biggest revelation was that I was really, really, really bored. I was bored with dieting for eighteen years – and actually putting on thirty pounds in the process. I was bored with not being able to stick to something that I wanted so much. I was bored with being a grown-up who wasn't able to control herself. I was bored with putting things off. I was bored with imagining how life would be better if I lost weight. I was bored with not being able to wear what I wanted. I was bored with always imagining the future, when I would be at so-and-so's wedding, looking great – and it never happening. I was bored with seeing my amazing friend Ruth never eating her child's leftovers – when I couldn't stop hoovering them up. I was bored with failing.

I was brought up by two schoolteachers, who were big on the ethos of learning, so being bored just wasn't part of the deal. And even now, saying 'I'm bored' makes me feel guilty. But that is what I felt. I'm a pretty intelligent person. I got ten O levels, five A levels, a degree, and a diploma in landscape photography. I have an amazing family and friends who I like being with a lot. I have a house that makes me happy when I walk through the front door and is filled with nice things. I'm achieving most of what I want in my career. My husband makes me laugh and is lovely. He and my daughter are the loves of my life. But I can't bloody stick to a diet. WHY?

Okay, so here is my small moment of epiphany after feeling this overwhelming boredom with myself. Imagine this:

I am at home again in the evening, one month into the diet, and I'm literally about to eat a three-cheese pizza. I believe this pizza is what will make me happy. When I dial the delivery number it's like I'm not consciously doing it. I'm on autopilot. I just have a need for pizza. I'm not happy. I'm not sad either. I just want my lovely pizza. Even as I eat my pizza I am thinking to myself that I shouldn't have it. But I do.

I'm watching **The House of Tiny Tearaways** *and the quite extraordinary Dr Tanya Byron is working closely with a young mum and dad and their two young children. They are sitting around a table and one of the kids is refusing to eat anything at all apart from yogurt, and is throwing the fit of the century. Scary stuff, to see the child so irate and the parents so helpless. As Tanya unravels the problem, it turns out that the mother can't have any more kids and is sad about that, and also underneath it all she doesn't want her children to grow up. She's happy with the baby stage and wants the children to have everything they want. Tanya tells the parents that this extreme eating disorder is really nothing to do with the child but is all up to the parents. Until the mother makes the decision that 'THIS IS IT, little Johnny is going to be a normal little boy and eat properly,' then nothing is going to change. The boy is getting away with it because HE CAN. Tanya tells his mother that she has to be 100 per cent totally sure that this is what she wants, and to change her focus, accepting no excuses; not caving in to the easy route and allowing the boy to do what he wants. Instead, she must make a decision and stick to it. Without that decision nothing will change. It is pure mind over matter stuff: if she sticks to it and is strong then her life will get so much easier.*

The transformation was unbelievable and extremely quick. Once he was faced with no get-out clause and a mother who was determined to change things, the little boy transformed his eating and the pasty look on his face disappeared almost immediately.

I am sitting eating my pizza and for some reason the programme has totally struck a chord with me.

*Beside the television is a rack full of fashion magazines, and I love to look at the clothes I don't believe I'll ever be able to buy but really hope one day I'll fit into. But I'm eating pizza. Helpless. Unable to control myself. It is like there are two parts of me. I want to be slim (my heart), but I want to eat what I want (my head). So I eat the pizza. But as I do, I suddenly come to realize that maybe **this is not about what goes into your mouth. It is about what goes on in your mind.** That little boy could eat healthily, just like I can if I decide that is what I'm going to do.*

Think about the split second between doing it and not doing it. Those precious moments of looking at a cake and deciding whether you are going to eat it or not eat it . . . It's your decision. It's your brain and your thoughts that will either get you through this or not.

There is this whole level of discussion going on under the surface all the time. But the truth is, there's no magic formula, and no time for discussion, either. Over a period of time I have had to teach my brain new tricks. I've had to outwit it and think two steps ahead of it. Miss Marple would be proud.

We are what we think. We think – then we do it. This may sound like psychobabble but it is true.

The lazy part of the brain that tells you not to bother – that niggling voice that tells you it's okay to eat the cake – I don't want to waste any more time listening to it. Nor do you.

But what do you do? How do you stop all the rubbish going on in your head?

First of all, you have to make a decision that you're going to do this. And nothing is going to stop you. You have to grab yourself by the scruff of the neck . . . I AM GOING TO DO THIS ONCE AND FOR ALL AND NOTHING IS GOING TO STAND IN MY WAY.

Accept that your head is trying to rule your heart and be strong. Battle with your subconscious niggles and win. Maybe your mind tells you, 'You can't stick to your diet. You have never done it before . . . why would you do it now. Have those chips over there.' Realize that it is your mind telling you this and you can say no to it. Because you are in charge.

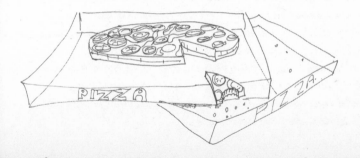

Tell yourself, 'I don't want those chips because I want to lose weight. I'm bored with my situation always being one where I'm not happy with myself. From now on I'm going to change my situation.'

Think through properly what eating that chip will mean to you : chips = not sticking to my diet = going off my diet = failing = eating more = putting on more weight = feeling worse about myself and unable to do what I want and feel the way I want.

You have to give yourself a strict talking to.

What do you really want in your life? Make a decision. Stick to it.

NOW WRITE IT DOWN AND PUT IT IN YOUR PURSE.

My bit of paper has two things that make me immediately focus on the decision I've made.

> I Want to be
> Fit, Fit, Fit.
>
> I WANT TO WEAR
> Size 12 Jeans.

The first bit is from a kids' programme called *Boogie Beebies*. Whenever that song comes on my daughter jumps up and sings it and does the actions. So it makes me think of her as well. And the bit about jeans may sound superficial but I just want to wear nice jeans. India and I are looking for the perfect jeans to reward ourselves with.

Look at your bit of paper every time you're troubled by food. Look at it and think about what you're doing. It may sound over the top, but who cares? It will work if you want it to. You can do it. India and I did it. And we're still doing it – every day.

India's Secret for Being Little Miss Sunshine

This is entirely subjective, and I apologize if it sounds smug given Neris's *cri de coeur* above, but it worked for me. After the first few days were over, and after I'd stopped feeling strange, which was on the morning of Day Six, I stopped thinking about being on a diet. Unless I was with Neris, when obviously we'd discuss what we were doing and how we were getting on in microscopic detail, I just got on with my everyday life. I treated dieting rather like I'd treat going to the hairdresser's to have a radical change of colour: it would take a few days to get used to it, but after that I wouldn't constantly be thinking, 'Oh my goodness, I have red hair now.' My hair would just be my hair. In the same manner, the way I ate just became the way I ate. Not eating carbs simply became what I did. This has made the diet very, very easy for me to follow. It's not a diet, to me. It's how I eat. And I eat really well (I'm writing this just having had crispy courgette rosti for lunch). My family eats what I eat, with mash or rice or pasta on the side. It's not a big deal.

How We Felt on Day Eleven
India: Up.
Neris: Down.

Phase One Day Twelve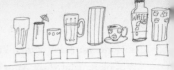

The usual. Water. Supplements. Breakfast. Walk.

You know how yesterday we were saying that people might be commenting on you looking somehow better? That's today's topic. First of all, don't be depressed if those comments haven't yet come your way. They will. But one of the incredibly frustrating things about dieting is that sometimes you feel and see a dramatic difference in the way you look – and you know you're not hallucinating, because your scales or tape measure back you up – and yet there is a distinct and demoralizing failure to notice on the part of the people around you. It makes you feel like grabbing a marker pen and writing 'I'm ten pounds down, actually!' in capital letters across your forehead. The truth of the matter is that the usual pattern, at least for us, is that you get the odd 'You're looking well,' and then nothing for a while, and then a sudden avalanche of 'My god, you've lost so much weight.' (Happily, the people you sleep with on a regular basis are usually a little bit quicker on the uptake, which is cheering.)

We touched on the subject of unhelpful friends much earlier in this book, but we think it's a topic that's worth revisiting. If you remember, we mentioned the 'friends' who said, 'You look fantastic, you don't need to lose any more,' when we weighed a hefty fifteen stone. Whether you're doing this diet in private, as we suggested, or in public, the comments may start any time round about now. And you need to be braced for them. As we've said before, there are people who may love you dearly but who aren't entirely at ease with the idea that trusty, reliably fat you is in the process of morphing into something unknown, i.e. something less reliably comfortable, or indeed comforting.

A great number of people – and we're sorry to say that when we say 'people' we mean 'women friends' – have serious difficulties with that concept. It may be that, as the designated fat friend, you're their excuse to pig out every now and then. The unlovely thought process behind this is, 'Well, she doesn't watch her weight, or care that she's fat, so if I have this chocolate cake with her, she's not going to make me feel bad about it. Besides, how could she? She's the size of a house.' By removing that possibility, since you're not eating chocolate cake any more, you're also removing your friend's excuse to binge. And that's quite likely to really piss her off, whether it's at a conscious or a subconscious level.

We're not saying it's an enormous deal, but we are telling you to be aware of it, and to get wise to it. When this friend suggests you go off the diet for a night, and join her for dinner, with pints of Baileys and a bag of chips on the way home afterwards, she isn't thinking about you; she is thinking about herself. Know this, and you've got the winning hand. Fall for it – thinking, she's my friend, she cares about me – and you've lost. Of course your friends care about you. But a lot of women also care quite a lot about their self-image, and as the fat friend you are an integral part of it.

The long and the short of it is that by losing weight you are going to look better, and by looking better you are going to make some people feel threatened. When I (India) was very overweight, nobody (mercifully) ever called me fat to my face, but I had a reply ready in my head – for decades – just in case. It was, 'At least I can go on a diet. What are you going to do – have a face and body transplant?' Childish, I know, but it cheered me up to know that I had a riposte if I was ever to be aggressed by one of those horse-faced twigs who assume that everybody would really rather look like them. Thin I can deal with; pinched and lollipop-headed, no thanks. And there are an awful lot of women around who equate physical beauty with near-anorexia. We hope you're not one of them – we like pretty faces better than spindly arms. But those spindly women aren't going to like you for losing weight and, by so doing, becoming prettier. We're not suggesting they're your closest girlfriends, obviously (and if they are, please get yourselves some new ones, pronto). They may be your boss, or a colleague, or the friend of a friend, or whatever. They exist in quite considerable numbers.

So, What to do About Them?

Ignore them. However, this is much easier said than done.
If it is your misfortune to sit opposite someone at work who
has an almost forensic interest in what you do and don't put in
your mouth, things can get very trying. In which case: be blunt.
We know we said to try to diet on the sly, but that can become
impossible if you've got Sherlock bloody Holmes on your back
for ten hours a day. Either be polite and say, 'I'm watching what
I eat,' or be impolite and loudly say (smiling), 'Do you have
food issues? Because I find your interest in what I eat obsessive
and weird.'

If that doesn't work, or if it sparks off World War Three –
always a possibility – play the same game. For every 'Oh, you're
eating ham and cheese again,' come back with 'And I see you're
gorging on chocolate for the third time today.' If your colleague
comments on your snack of nuts, comment (unfavourably) on
her snack of crisps.

Force her to pay you a compliment. Hold out your trousers
and say, 'Look, my waistband's become really loose.' She'll
hardly be able to deny it.

If anyone tells you that low-carbing is unhealthy, refer back
to pages 66–8. Or laugh out loud: who's healthier – the person
having grilled salmon and salad for lunch, or the one chomping
down on a lard-burger and fries?

Being honest is a good policy, too. If you're offered
something you know you can't eat, say, 'I'm doing so well today,
I'm feeling pleased with myself, and I don't want to spoil it,
so no thanks.'

If you genuinely feel hurt by a comment ('Bloody hell!
You've put on so much weight!'), then say so. 'That's not a
terribly helpful remark,' you can say, which puts the ball back
in their court.

Neris is a big fan of love-bombing. If someone makes a
remark you don't like, bombard him or her with insanely
positive things. Instead of acting hurt, say, 'You're so lucky to
have such a beautiful figure.' Heap compliments on their lovely

shiny hair, or nice clear skin, or beautiful hands, or whatever. It will take them by surprise and throw them off guard. They've been bitchy to you, but you've been heavenly back, and now they're confused. And you feel mighty fine.

If all else fails, tell them to fuck off.

Be aware, though, that the nightmare friend/boss/ colleague scenario outlined above is quite an extreme example – though food does make people behave in extreme ways. Also be on your guard for the more subtle forms of sabotage that come from closer friends. A good, non-aggressive but guilt-inducing line to have at the ready is, 'I'm very good at sabotaging myself. I don't need your help.'

Here's a similar situation from Neris's journal:

Some 'slim friends who like to see people eat' came to see me and they were really on at me about being on a diet and it being a fad. They kept trying to get me to eat what they were eating but I resisted.

How, I don't know! Actually it was sheer bloody mindedness and the fact that I really need to have a good day behind me now where I get on with everything. I need to remember that you have to be careful with some people. They don't always have your best interests at heart.

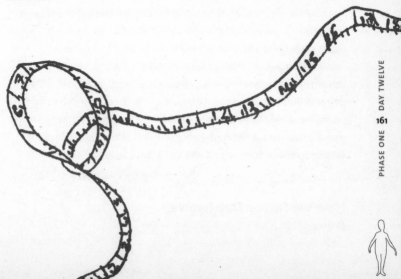

I was having dinner at my friend's house. She knows I'm low-carbing, but she cooked pasta for starters and potato gratin to accompany the main course, and then there was pudding. I felt very embarrassed, and had the smallest possible quantities of food I shouldn't have eaten at all. But I couldn't not eat – it would have been so rude. Right?

Well, congratulations on having nice manners. But no, it's not right. You should have passed on the pasta, and had the meat and vegetables but not the potato. At pudding time, you could have said, 'I don't suppose you have any cheese lurking in your fridge?' If you'd done this, chances are your friend would have smacked herself theatrically on the forehead, and loudly exclaimed, for everyone else to hear, 'Oh God, I forgot, YOU'RE ON A DIET.' We don't blame you for wanting to avoid this scenario. But you have to decide what matters more: your ten seconds of embarrassment, or your weight loss. Besides, you hear those words and mentally add, 'BECAUSE YOU'RE SUCH A GIANT FAT HEFFALUMP', and feel anxious and humiliated in advance. But you know, the other people sitting at that table wouldn't have added those crazy words, or sniggered, or thought to themselves, 'Yeah, she looks like she could do with going on a diet, the big fat hog.' They'd have been admiring. We know, because we really admired people who had the self-control to look after their weight – and we admired them doubly for sticking to their guns in social situations.

Whether your friend cooked a carby meal accidentally-on-purpose or whether it was a genuine oversight, people don't ask people round to dinner to stuff them with food – they ask them round because they enjoy their company. Be good company. Don't make a fuss about not being able to eat certain things: just eat what you're allowed to eat, and enjoy yourself.

How We Felt on Day Twelve

Better.

Phase One Day Thirteen

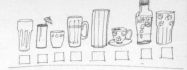

Bravo! You've only got today and tomorrow to go, and then Phase One is over.

OR IS IT ?

Today – following water, supplements and breakfast, naturally – we want you to spend your walking time having a little think.

It's time to be honest. Brutally so. If you feel you've followed the diet to the letter, consider yourself garlanded with laurels, skip the rest of this chapter, and have a nice day.

Still reading? Hmm. Okay. So we're assuming you've cheated.

Don't despair. It doesn't mean you're doomed to failure. Flip forwards a couple of days and read Neris's journal entries for proof. She was the queen of cheating – but she didn't come clean about it for a good long while. Of course, it was only when she was able to look her cheating in the eye that the weight started really coming off. There's trying to diet, and there's lying to yourself about succeeding. Neris knows all about this.

We'd meet for lunch and talk about the diet, and I'd say, 'I'm so pleased, I weigh such-and-such at the moment,' and she'd say, 'That's great! So do I.' And – I'm sure she'll forgive me for writing this – it was transparently obvious to me that, give or take the odd pound or two, she looked identical to how she'd looked a fortnight previously. And yet here she was claiming to have lost half a stone. It made me feel very confused, for a while. She was wearing the same clothes, and they fitted her the same way – so where was the weight loss she was claiming had made her so delighted? I've never known Neris lie about anything in all the time I've known her – she is a realist, not a fantasist. And yet here she was – every time we met up – claiming to have lost weight when she clearly hadn't. She also perfected quite a nifty trick, which was to stand up, beam, and say, 'Can you tell I've lost weight?' When it's put like that, it's very very hard to say, 'Er, no.'

So, yeah. We know about lying to yourself. We know about sticking to the diet all day and then ordering a pizza and wolfing it down and pretending it hasn't happened. We know about the two bottles of wine that seem to have found their way down your gullet when you weren't looking. We know about the chocolate bars that somehow fail to register if you're keeping a food diary with fitday.com. Here's Neris, writing once she'd got over her cheaty phase:

I'm scared to admit failure. I want to succeed but I've got the ghosts of old – failed – diets weighing down my neck, and that means that sometimes I'm not quite brave enough to be completely honest. Did I really just have a bit of bread? Nah. It was only in my mouth for second. Does that count? And will anyone notice that I just had too much of that cheese?

Believe me when I say that I've been in denial for years. Sometimes I would speak to India and for some reason just tell her that I was sticking to it and that it was going great. I have talked to friends and said I was on a diet, and gone home and eaten a ton of carbs. I know what it's like to lie about it. And I was lying to myself. I'm not leading people up the garden path for no reason. I know what the reason is. It is that I literally can't be honest with myself. I am too scared to admit that I can't stick to something I want to do. I've sat in Weight Watchers classes in the past and sworn blind that I have stuck to their diet all week. I've done food diaries for nutritionists and amended the contents so it would say what I thought they would want to see.

But it is all rubbish. The only way I have been able to stop doing this is just to be completely straightforward and say, 'I ate that bit of bread because I felt sad and nothing else would satisfy my needs.' When you can admit that, you're getting somewhere. You have to be completely up front. Good or bad. You are what you are, and you have to stop beating yourself up and just say the truth: I ate that because I wanted to. At a certain point I had to get real. You have to get real. You are overweight because you eat too much. Honesty is the only thing that will get you through.

And that's why today is designated honesty day. Please reply honestly to the following questions.

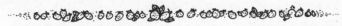

Have you been drinking your water?
You know, we don't make this stuff up off the tops of our heads. The knowledge we have gained is first-hand. We've done the diet. We know what works. When we say you have to drink your water, we mean it. Drink your flipping water. It's speeding up the weight-loss process. It's flushing out toxins and the less desirable by-products of this way of eating, which means that the water is being kind to your kidneys. It's really, really good for your skin. It stops you being constipated. It makes you feel full. If we don't drink enough water, our weight loss slows down. Yours will too. Just blimmin' drink it.

Have you been reading the labels?
You've got to. You can't just close your eyes and hope for the best. If that ready meal has starch and sugar in it, it can mean you're eating quadruple the amount of carbs you're allowed for the whole day in the space of one meal. If you regularly eat ready-cooked food – and even if you only use them occasionally – ALWAYS READ THE LABEL. And don't think, it won't hurt just this once. It will. It has.

Have you been snacking on forbidden things?
Tell the truth. As we have been saying until we're blue in the face, you can't cheat at this stage of the diet. It's an absolute deal-breaker. You may have snuck in a few biscuits or a couple of slices of cake – or even something really small-seeming, like a couple of roast potatoes – and 'forgotten' about it. Well, don't forget. It's derailing you.

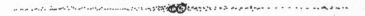

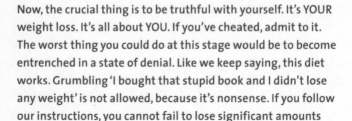

Have you been snacking on specific forbidden things in the belief that they're somehow 'healthy'?

We are rolling our eyes. Just because you found that cereal bar in the health food shop doesn't mean it's an aid to weight loss. Just because you've had a bowl of low-calorie cereal instead of the old Crunchy Nuts doesn't make AN IOTA of difference on this way of eating. Ditto organic biscuits versus bog-standard, or sugar-free jam versus ordinary. If it's not on the list, you aren't allowed to eat it. Full stop.

Have you been skipping meals to make up for cheating?

No, no, no, no. You can't skip meals. It's one of the golden rules. If you skip meals, your body holds on to its fat stores, simple as that. You need to eat three square meals a day and supplement them with as many snacks as you feel the need for.

Now, the crucial thing is to be truthful with yourself. It's YOUR weight loss. It's all about YOU. If you've cheated, admit to it. The worst thing you could do at this stage would be to become entrenched in a state of denial. Like we keep saying, this diet works. Grumbling 'I bought that stupid book and I didn't lose any weight' is not allowed, because it's nonsense. If you follow our instructions, you cannot fail to lose significant amounts of weight.

PHASE ONE · DAY THIRTEEN

But anyway, okay, you cheated. You ate things you weren't supposed to eat. It's not all bad: you still probably weigh less than you did a fortnight ago, though your weight loss has not been in any way dramatic, and you probably don't feel that great – because your body doesn't know whether it's coming or going. You know what you have to do now: get back in the saddle. Flip back to Day One and start again. Please try to do this only once – as we have already said, neither this diet nor your body much likes stopping and starting. Muck around for long enough, and your body will feel like it's under siege, and hold on to its reserves of fat. That would be the opposite of a result.

Do not attempt to move on to Phase Two if you've been cheating. It won't work. Go back to the beginning, and start again. It's only two more weeks out of your life. And you'll thank us in the end.

It might help to re-read the whole of this book until now. Really read it. Ask yourself questions. Absorb information. Get yourself in the right frame of mind. There is nothing unique about you, and that means there is absolutely no reason why you should fail – even if you weigh 400 pounds. The past is the past. Forget about it. Tomorrow is the future. And your future is thin. You deserve it. It's within grasp. Now, go for it.

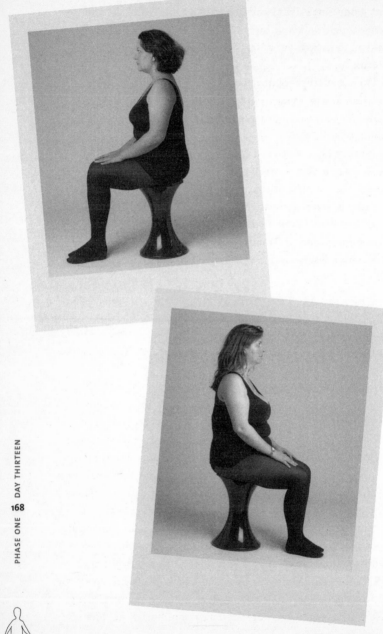

Phase One Day Fourteen

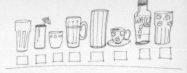

You've made it! How brilliant is that? We take our hats off and throw them in the air, whooping with delight on your behalf.

You're looking and feeling miles better. Your clothes are getting looser by the day. You may even have dumped those horrible tent-dresses and gone to the shops to buy something more fitted (one of the great, great joys of this diet for us was when we could suddenly wander into any High Street shop and buy clothes – not stretchy clothes, or things made of cotton jersey, but real, proper clothes, in real, proper sizes).

Congratulations. We really mean it. We know how far you've come, just as we know that the whole process may have been a bit up and down emotionally. But we hope you're now firmly entrenched. We hope you've got the bug. Now, a confession. We lost five stone each. Obviously, we didn't do this in two weeks. It took us a year. And this is what we did: we repeated Phase One for several months – six, to be precise.

Now, you're either thinking, 'You've got to be joking,' or you're thinking, 'Okaaaay . . . I can live with that.' Your reaction will determine what you do next. If you didn't have that much weight to lose to start with – two stone, say – move on to Phase Two tomorrow. If you have more than that to lose, do consider staying on Phase One for a while longer. How much longer? Only you can tell. We suggest moving to Phase Two when your goal weight is within reach – say when it's a stone away. Things slow down very slightly on Phase Two, and you have to ask yourself whether you're happy for that to happen in exchange for a broader menu and a wider variety of things to eat.

However, if you do decide to stay on Phase One – and really, you could stay on it indefinitely if you were so inclined – we're going to allow you alcohol. From tomorrow, you may drink DRY white wine, red wine and champagne (not all at once!). Better still, develop a taste for vodka, and have it with either diet tonic or with soda water and a twist of fresh lime. This equals zero carbs.

Whatever your decision, pour yourself a drink. Cheers! You've achieved an amazing thing.

Time to buy a full-length mirror, if you don't own one already.

The Stakes

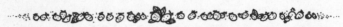

Neris:

▸ I wanted to buy nice underwear.

▸ I wanted to wear V-shaped T-shirts at the gym, not old baggy crappy ones.

▸ I wanted people to notice more weight loss and I wanted more compliments.

▸ I want to lose my tummy fold.

India:

▸ I wanted more compliments too – they became addictive.

▸ I wanted to look hot in a swimsuit.

▸ I wanted my stomach to shrink more.

▸ I wanted to buy smaller bras.

What are your stakes?

Write them down here.

_____

_____

_____

_____

_____

_____

_____

_____

_____

_____

_____

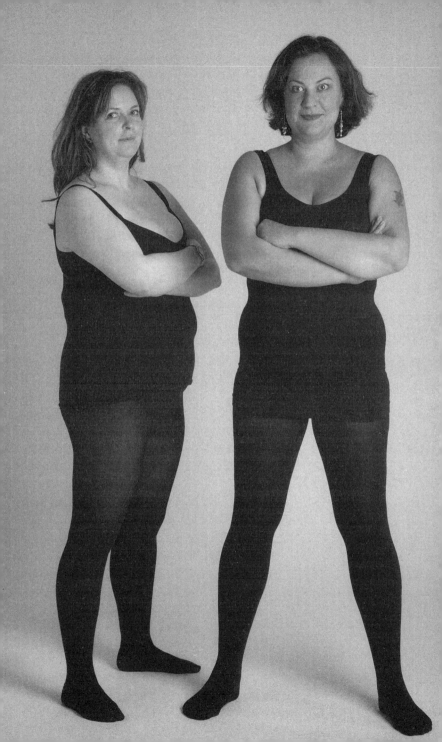

Part Three
The Diet – Phase Two

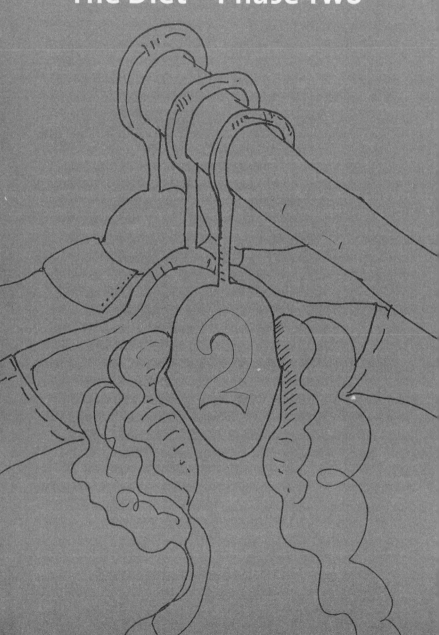

Phase Two Week One

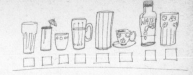

Once again, congratulations. You may be coming to this part of the diet after only a fortnight, or it may have taken you several weeks or months (as was the case for us) to get here. Either way, welcome, and well done. Please weigh yourself again before commencing Phase Two, and take your measurements again (see page 72).

So what happens now? Well, you still need to watch your carbs, obviously. Low-carbing, as we said earlier in the book, is a way of eating that is for life. But we're now going to take you away from the restrictive confines of Phase One, and broaden out your eating quite dramatically over the coming weeks.

To recap: this is basically what you have been eating so far:

- All meats, including hams, bacon, pâtés and salamis
- Eggs
- Green leafy vegetables
- Many other veg, provided they're not starchy
- Fish and shellfish
- Cheese
- Nuts
- Double cream
- Butter and peanut butter
- Olive oil
- Groundnut oil
- Olives
- Tofu
- Soya milk
- Whey protein powder
- Splenda sugar substitute
- Lemons and limes

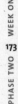

That list is still valid, and will still be the bedrock of most of your meals. However, we're going to add to it. In Phase Two you will also be allowed:

▸ Non-leafy green vegetables – onions, for instance – in increased quantities
▸ All the berries – blueberries, raspberries, strawberries, etc.
▸ Cantaloupe and honeydew melon
▸ Seeds, as well as nuts
▸ Dark chocolate
▸ Coconut milk
▸ Plain yogurt
▸ Alcohol (hooray!)
▸ Soya flour – which means you can now bake (double hooray!)
▸ Ground linseed – ditto
▸ Stone-ground, wholewheat bread

All of the above need to be eaten in moderation. In moderation. In moderation. Once more: in moderation. That means twice a week to start off with. Otherwise you will be thrown off-course in a spectacular way.

Furthermore, Phase Two allows you – eventually, not straight away – to fall off the wagon occasionally. Given that you're going to be eating this way for the rest of your life, we don't expect you to be saintly at all times. This is not, however, a licence to slip up: going off-piste at Christmas is one thing; doing it weekly is another. And anyway, there's no need to do it weekly – or at all – when you can now have chocolate mousse for pudding, provided you're happy to use Splenda. A celebratory evening menu might look something like this:

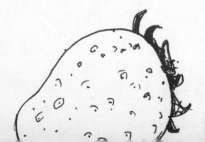

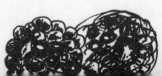

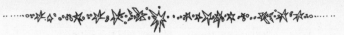

STEAMED CLAMS IN GARLIC AND HERB BUTTER

**FILLET OF BEEF WITH BÉARNAISE SAUCE
ROCKET AND PARMESAN SALAD, GREEN BEANS AND ROAST
TOMATOES**

RASPBERRY PAVLOVA

CHEESE

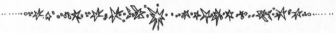

Hardly unbearably strict, we think you'll agree. In fact, almost crazily fabulous. And not something you'd feel shy about serving to non-dieters, either.

Now, we're not going to add all of the above new foods in one fell swoop, because that would clearly have disastrous results. Your body needs time, and plenty of it, to adjust to each new food – and bear in mind it'll adjust much more happily if you eat the new food with some fat. We're not going to lie to you: you will be able to eat these things in moderation, and from time to time, but not at every meal. While having scrambled eggs on toast every once in a while is one thing, sitting down to a mound of buttered toast every morning is always going to be a disaster. You're going to have to make some choices, but don't worry: we'll be there to guide you through them.

We'll work our way through the new foods in this order:

▸ Alcohol – because we think you deserve it (if you don't drink, move down the list)

▸ Dark chocolate (ditto if you don't like chocolate)

▸ Porridge oats

▸ Soya flour and ground linseed

▸ Extra vegetables in increased quantities.

▸ Coconut milk

▸ Berries

▸ Melons, and other summer fruit

- Seeds
- Plain yogurt
- Wholewheat, stone-ground bread

In the final phase of the diet, we will reintroduce:
- Other fruits
- Legumes
- Starchy veg
- Whole grains (i.e. brown things, not white)

But don't even think about these four items for the time being. We're just letting you know for future reference.

The idea is to introduce one new thing at a time and give it a week to see how it goes, and how it impacts on your metabolism. Your scales, and the way you're feeling, will be able to tell you all you need to know. If you bloat instantly and feel like you're bursting out of your clothes upon reintroducing wheat, for instance, learn from it. We're against people believing they're allergic to everything all the time, but in the case of wheat there does seem to be cause for concern.

If you work through everything on the list too fast, you will put on weight. So don't. Take your time. You're still on a diet, and you still want to lose weight. If you feel one week isn't enough to gauge whether one particular food agrees with you or not, give it two weeks.

Having said that, we believe it is enormously cheering to reintroduce alcohol and chocolate in the same week (but for heaven's sake not at the same time, please – it's hard to keep control of how much chocolate you're eating if you have a couple of glasses of wine inside you). So, go ahead. At some stage today, pour yourself a drink.

You may reintroduce the first nine items on the above list in any order you like, provided it's one at a time, each for a period of one week (or two). Leave the bread until last. For the purposes of this book, we're following the numerical order as it is above, so it may be easier if you do too. But if you desperately crave berries above alcohol, then go right ahead and have berries first. They'll taste amazing, by the way – almost unimaginably sweet.

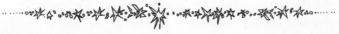

Alcohol

When you say alcohol, do you mean any drink at all?
No. Not any drink at all, at all. You need to know two things: the first is that spirits have zero carbs – that's 'clean' spirits, 'hard liquor', rather than the sugar-laden ones such as Southern Comfort or Bailey's, which are and always will be completely forbidden. So don't even go there. (A pina colada, for example, has thirty-two grams of carb per serving – which is, freakily, more than you've been eating in a whole day during Phase One.)

But you can have gin, vodka, rum and whisky. Our tipple of choice is vodka, the cleanest spirit of all, and – we find – the least hangover-inducing. (Beware of hangovers, by the way. If you've been following our instructions and not drinking for the past fortnight – or more – then go easy with the alcohol. One drink is usually plenty to start off with. India went to a wedding a week into Phase Two, had three glasses of wine over two hours, and had to leave to throw up. Gross but true. So pace yourself, and don't forget your water.)

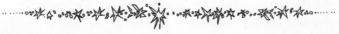

Mixers

Mixers, as you are no doubt aware, are awash with sugar. My (India's) pet hate, Diet Coke, is awash with appalling amounts of artificial sugars, and we're not talking relatively safe Splenda. It's also awash with monstrous amounts of additives and chemicals, which have no part to play whatsoever in this way of eating. Do you know, everyone I know who has a weight problem is addicted to this stuff – and none of them think it's bad for them, or a contributing factor in any way, because it's 'diet', innit? I say, DO NOT DRINK DIET COKE. Always remember, you are not following a calorie-controlled diet,

which means that 'diet' products are irrelevant. Actually they're
worse than irrelevant – they are actively NO GOOD. They are
evil. They have horns and a tail.

Quite aside from anything else, Diet Coke's artificial
sweeteners alone can stall weight loss indefinitely in a great
number of people. You have been warned.

By the same token, don't drink Irn-Bru, Fanta, Sprite, or
any of those sweet, sugary, rubbish-laden drinks – even if they
are the 'diet' version. Ditto lemonade, limeade, lime cordial
(or any cordial: they're primarily sugar). Ditto fruit juice of any
description. Cranberry juice may be great if you have cystitis,
but it's full of sugar. Orange juice is also full of sugar, plus it's
horribly acidic.

So, what does that leave you with? Soda water or diet tonic.
Of these, soda water is the best, though diet tonic isn't the end
of the world (and is the only exception to our rule about not
eating or drinking anything 'diet', ever). If that feels bland, add
a slice of lemon or a squirt of lime juice (not cordial). We won't
lie to you; we had to train ourselves to develop a taste for vodka
and soda. At first, it seemed awfully bland. Now, we love it.
There's a reason why vodka, soda and fresh lime is the models'
drink of choice.

You may also drink wine of either colour, red (two carbs
per glass) being marginally preferable than white (one carb,
but none of the known benefits of drinking red wine in
moderation). If you're going to drink white wine, it's got to be
dry: if your tipple of choice is Gewürztraminer, you're going
to have to bite the bullet. Champagne is okay in moderation,
meaning two glasses.

And please remember: being allowed alcohol doesn't mean
you now have to go and drink excessively every night. Drinking
in moderation doesn't stall anyone that we've come across.
Drinking loads does. This is because your body will burn
alcohol for fuel when it's available before it burns your own fat.
Do bear this in mind: every drink, even if it's carb-free, means
a small delay. Small delays we can live with. Big ones, not.

Chocolate

Now, on to chocolate. You can only have the dark stuff, with the highest cocoa content possible, and you can only have it in moderation. By 'moderation', we mean a square or two a day. If you think you don't like dark chocolate, think again. If you've been following Phase One properly, it will taste sweet and delicious. If it doesn't, cook with it – add Splenda if you're okay with it – and make things like chocolate mousse (NOT every day! Once a week, tops!).

On with the first day of Phase Two, then. You know the drill: Water. Supplements. Breakfast. Walk. Today, we'd like you to increase your walk by an extra fifteen minutes. We would also like you to think about upping your exercise. Don't panic: it's not imminent. But do have a think about what you might find bearable: yoga, pilates, the dreaded gym, swimming, whatever. This isn't because we're mean. It's because we don't want you to sag.

See previous entries for lunch and supper ideas, if you still need them: we hope that by now you're into the groove and understand that the easiest way to eat is by adapting your own family recipes.

If we were you, we'd save the alcohol until tonight, and don't forget to keep the chocolate and alcohol separate – you don't want to get tiddly and consume a family-size bar. Before we go, one last thing: congratulations again for getting to this stage.

The structure of the book changes from here onwards: what you now do is introduce the new food of your choice on a Monday, and carry on eating that way all week. Watch your body. Weigh yourself the following Monday. If the weight is still falling off, great – though please note that, with the reintroduction of more carbs, it will slow down a little. If it stalls altogether, first of all remember that weight loss is not linear and that it is entirely normal, in Phase Two, to lose nothing for a couple of weeks – or longer, but not more than four weeks – and then suddenly drop a load almost overnight. If the new food causes you to put on weight, even eaten in moderation, drop it immediately.

So this week, for instance, you will be eating everything you were eating in Phase One, plus alcohol (but see above for restrictions) and a limited amount of chocolate. You will still start the day with water, supplements and breakfast, and you will still be going for your walk which should, from today, take a minimum of thirty minutes. Carry on for the week; we'll see you again in Week Two.

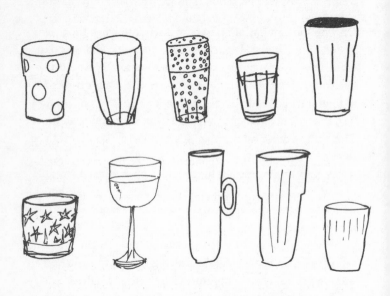

Phase Two Week Two

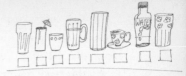

Hello again. We hope you've had a nice week and not too many hangovers. And we hope you've managed to be intelligent about the chocolate, and not indulged in any crazy choco-binges. If you've found the reintroduction of chocolate difficult to manage, i.e. if you've had any trouble at all with controlling the amount you eat, now is the time to be honest with yourself, do yourself a favour, and ration it properly: have it only on Friday nights, or – if it's proving to be a complication too far – stop having it for the time being. Bear in mind that I (India) am writing this from the point of view of someone who doesn't have a sweet tooth, and who is perfectly happy nibbling at one square of dark chocolate a few times a week. You may be different. If you are, know it, and do something about it. Take control. You've been dieting for weeks, with great results – don't chuck it all away because your cravings for chocolate have returned, big time. This applies to all of the foods we'll be reintroducing. If you find yourself eating them excessively and can't seem to control your appetite for them, chuck them off the list. Life's too short to get fat again.

Neris wrote in her journal about chocolate:

Compelled to go to garage to buy a paper and a chocolate bar. Don't know what it is but this has been a combination that fits me and it is a difficult one to break. I am driving to the garage. Not feeling particularly bad or good, just focused on needing a little bit of chocolate.

Just called India from the forecourt . . . she has talked me into having dark chocolate. Really not as nice and satisfying, I'm sure, as milk chocolate . . . I know it is a lot better for me and it still is chocolate (I suppose). I'm going in to get some. They don't have any! There is a gap where it says Green and Black but they have all gone. Crisis. What do I do now?

I need a bit of chocolate. Call India again. She's talked me down. And now she says I need to drink some water . . . from my bottle.

Uuhhhhhh so boring. I've done it. It works for a few moments. I've got to distract myself. I'm beginning to get strange looks from the people at the garage.

I'm going in to look at a slimming magazine and get inspiration. All the time drinking my water . . . okay . . . panic over.

Rest of the day stuck to it.

Now, weigh and measure yourself. Do this every Monday.

Porridge oats

This week we are introducing porridge – that's real porridge oats, not anything that's 'instant' or comes in microwaveable sachets. You are now allowed a small mugful of raw oats two mornings a week, three once you're exercising. (Not yet! Don't panic and see pages 206–10.) Tip the oats into a pan with double the quantity of liquid (soya milk, water or a mixture of both), simmer for ten minutes or so, and eat. You can add Splenda (or salt), vanilla extract, two chipped squares of dark chocolate, a glug of double cream, ground cinnamon, nuts, and so on. I like having it with cream, crushed cardamom seeds and the merest droplet of rosewater.

You may only have porridge once during twenty-four hours – i.e. don't have two bowlfuls in a day. We strongly suggest having it at the obvious time – first thing in the morning – and following it with your brisk walk immediately afterwards. Never have porridge after midday.

Don't forget: always try and eat fat with the new food. This lessens its impact on your blood sugar.

Think yourself slim

Neris and I found it very difficult to imagine ourselves slim. Or slimmer, even. It felt like a really delusional thing to do, to be standing in a department store ogling a skimpy dress or a pair of skinny jeans and thinking, 'One day soon, that piece of clothing is going to look great on me.' 'Yeah, right,' a part of my brain would pipe up. 'In your dreams, Fatty.' I have to say, Neris kept the faith to a greater extent than I ever managed: I remember one lunch when we met and she announced – being roughly a size twenty-two at the time – that she couldn't wait to be a size twelve.

Part of me greatly admired her – there is something very empowering, to use one of my least favourite words, about being so vocal about your ambitions: if you say it out loud, it's much harder to go back on your word.

Nevertheless, part of me also thought she was mad.

You are now getting to the stage where, having already experienced dramatic weight loss, the goal should be clearly visible, rather than pie (as it were) in the sky. Today, we want you to concentrate on visualizing yourself slim, even slimmer than you are now, at your dream weight. You may find this easy . . . or you may not. In which case, here is some stuff that we hope will be useful. Some of it's quite hippyish, I'm afraid. But it all helps.

Today's instruction is to get back in touch with your body, man. Seriously. It has been our misfortune (in a sense – in another it has been the most life-enhancing experience ever) to have spent considerable amounts of time in hospital wards full of very sick children. After the merest five minutes in such an environment, you become truly and pathetically grateful for the things you take for granted every single day: the fact that you can breathe without difficulty, and go to sleep at night without a canister of oxygen by your side. The fact that you can walk, run, skip, dance, without getting blue and tired within ten minutes. The fact that your limbs obey the commands from your brain; and the fact that the wiring in that brain works perfectly. The fact that you can talk and sing. That you can laugh. That you can move, and don't rely on someone pushing your wheelchair. That you are free, and happy, and not in pain. That your life expectancy is good, and that you are well. That all you have to worry about, as far as your body is concerned, is dropping some weight. Which you are doing.

Broaden it out: your amazing body may have borne you

amazing children, and it's easy to lose sight – especially if those children are now surly teenagers – of how utterly miraculous that was, and remains. Your body nourished those children, both inside the womb and out. Your body is your friend, at all times, and it works indescribably hard for you, every second of every minute of every day.

When you're overweight, it's incredibly easy to lose sight of all of this – especially if, like us, you reach a stage where looking down makes you feel uncomfortable (neither of us looked in a full-length mirror for about ten years). But now it's time to re-connect. Have a long, steady look at yourself. Every bit of you. Because every bit has a story to tell, and every bit – every scar, every dent, every wrinkle – is part of you. Never mind if you hate your upper arms, or your stomach, or your chin. It's all there, in working order, and working for you. We really want you to love yourself more with every day of Phase Two that passes. This is probably happening anyway, because with the dress sizes dropping and the large amounts of weight you've already lost, it would be difficult not to feel better about yourself. But we want you to love the inside of your body as well as the outside. We even want you to love your internal organs. Your lungs, your kidneys, your liver, your heart – they're all there, beavering away, keeping you well. So don't just love the new way your body looks. Love the way it works, too.

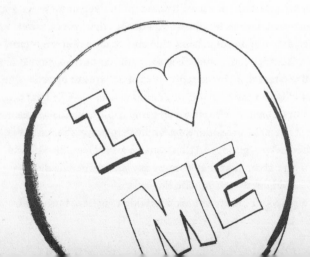

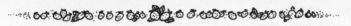

Here are some of the things you can look forward to eating during Phase Two:

▸ Pancakes made with soya flour, to which you can add berries
▸ Muffins made with soya flour, ditto – though savoury ones are pretty nice too
▸ Quiche with a soya-flour crust
▸ Crustless cheesecake
▸ Courgette chips
▸ 'Spaghetti' made using spaghetti squash, dressed with your favourite sauce
▸ Strawberries and cream
▸ Home-made chocolate truffles
▸ Deep-fried onion rings, using soya flour
▸ Brownies, made using soya flour and Splenda

And so on. The list is only as limited as your imagination.

As I (India) have mentioned before, I really like cooking. And I want to make it clear that even though you can create your own modified recipes, you can also use 'normal' cookbooks and create feasts based on this way of eating. We could give you dozens of recipes, but it's pointless, because you'll find dozens yourself – and besides, we're not professional chefs writing a cookbook. One of the things we dislike about diet books is the idea that you can only cook the (usually rather grim) recipes at the back. The opposite is true in our case – you can use whatever recipe you like, provided it adheres to our rules. You'd be surprised at the number that do.

So I thought I'd go through three cookbooks I often use to illustrate the truth of this. When I embarked on this way of eating, I was keen to order special low-carb cookbooks, and felt that I would probably never eat 'normal' food again. I was completely wrong. The low-carb cookbooks served their purpose, but I soon returned to Nigel, Nigella, et al., and I haven't looked back. Here's the proof:

From Annie Bell's *In My Kitchen*:

- Cocktail sausages with mustard dip
- Devils on horseback
- Quails' eggs with saffron salt
- Smoked salmon with keta
- Crudité dips
- Potted crab
- Prawns with chorizo and sherry
- Squid and tomato stew
- Mackerel rillettes
- Red peppers stuffed with Gorgonzola
- Portobello mushrooms wrapped in Parma ham
with goat's cheese
- Spinach soup with ricotta
- Chilled courgette soup
- Cheat's chicken Kiev
- Stuffed tomatoes
- Greek beef casserole with feta
- Kleftiko
- King prawns and mussels with basil purée
. . . and so on.

From Rose Gray and Ruth Rogers's *River Café Cook Book Easy*:

- Mozzarella and red pepper
- Green beans and anchovy
- Asparagus and anchovy
- Porcini and Parmesan
- Crab and fennel salad
- Beef carpaccio
- Roasted langoustine
- Roast whole squid
- Monkfish spiedini
- Grilled scallops
- Dover sole with capers
- Grilled tuna with fennel seeds
- Chicken with nutmeg

- ► Guinea fowl with fennel
- ► Roast quail with sage
- . . . and so on.

From Nigel Slater's *The Kitchen Diaries*:
- ► A salad of fennel, winter leaves and Parmesan
- ► A salad of winter cabbage and bacon
- ► Stew
- ► Clear, hot mussel soup
- ► Chicken patties with rosemary and pancetta
- ► Roast pumpkin, spicy tomato sauce
- ► Pork chops, mustard sauce
- ► English cheese salad
- ► Pork burgers with lime leaves and coriander
- ► Roast fillet of lamb with anchovy and mint
- ► Chicken with mushrooms and lemon grass
- ► Mackerel with cumin and lemon
- . . . and so on.

My point is, you don't need any special cookbooks to do this diet: what you have on your shelf will be ample, and will produce delicious meals that will delight everybody you feed them to (including your dear self), without giving anyone the impression that this is diet food. Which it isn't, you know. It's clean, healthy, home-cooked food that just happens to be low-carb.

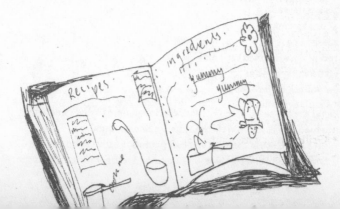

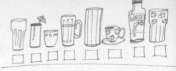

Phase Two Week Three

Water. Supplements. Breakfast. Walk. You know. Now weigh and measure yourself.

Soya Flour and Ground Linseed

This week we will be introducing soya flour and ground linseed (the latter has the advantage of being a known 'superfood'). Again, we're not going to go crazy and start our very own soya bakery. But we will be eating the flour/linseed in moderation. This means all sorts of things, primarily that you can now have pancakes for breakfast, and make low-carb 'bread'. If you've missed squidgy things over the past few weeks, your agony (except it wasn't that painful, was it?) is over. If you haven't missed squidgy things, congratulations: your palate is re-educating itself beautifully.

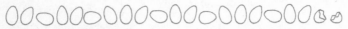

FAUX-WAFFLES/PANCAKES

You can get ground flaxseed (aka linseed) from your friends at the health food shop. If you try to do it yourself in a coffee grinder or blender, it won't be fine enough. Flaxseeds are very good, because of their high Omega 3 content.

40g ground flaxseed
60g walnut pieces
50g finely ground almonds
2 tsp ground cinnamon
1/4 tsp sea salt
4 tbsp Splenda
4 large eggs
240ml unsweetened soya milk
1 tsp baking powder
groundnut oil for frying

Blend the flaxseed, walnuts, almonds, cinnamon, salt and sweetener in a food processor until the walnuts are finely ground.

In a bowl, whisk the eggs and half (120ml) the soya milk. Add the walnut mixture and combine well. Cover and refrigerate for at least an hour, or overnight (but no longer).

When you're ready to eat, add baking powder and the remaining milk, then stir well.

Heat an oiled greased frying pan and drop blobs of the mixture on to it. This makes US-style fat pancakes, not crepes. Cook for about two minutes or until browned, then flip. You can have them slathered with butter, and you could also add vanilla extract to the batter.

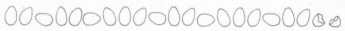

You are allowed two of these twice a week.

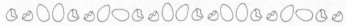

MICROWAVED LINSEED 'BREAD'

25g butter
2 medium eggs
4 heaped tbsp ground linseed
1 tsp baking powder

Melt the butter, let it cool a bit, add the eggs and mix. Add the linseed and baking powder. Mix again. Let it sit for a couple of minutes to thicken. Pour into a small microwaveable container (about 5 x 4 inches/12 x 10cm) and blast on full power for three minutes. Leave to cool for improved texture. You can also add cheese, bacon pieces, herbs or whatever.

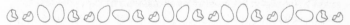

You are allowed two slices of this twice a week.

You will find many other recipes involving this week's foods on the net – we only mention this because neither of them crop up very often in ordinary cookery books. For more ways to use them, try looking up recipes on www.lowcarber.org, www.stellastyle.com or www.lowcarbluxury.com, to name but the tip of a most enormous iceberg. (Make sure you check out the before/after photographs, where applicable. We think we've done well, but some people lose literally hundreds of pounds eating this way and the photos are jaw-droppingly impressive.)

Building Your Confidence

From India's journal:

My mother made a remark about my having lost weight. A miracle of sorts, really – if she's noticed, it must really be showing.

We do hope you're feeling more physically confident. Today's exercise, now that you love your body more (we sincerely hope) is to build on that new-found confidence. Every woman needs a few tricks up her sleeve, and here are some of ours.

1. Don't throw away your Big Pants just yet. The temptation to go skipping about in micro-underwear is overwhelming (and this week is probably a good time to think about buying some), but frankly unless you're the size of Victoria Beckham (and we sincerely hope you're not dieting if you are that size – quasi-anorexic is not a great look!), then chances are there's always an occasion when Pants of Steel come in handy. So hang on to them – even if the time when you wore them every day has long passed. If they're falling off you, buy some new ones in a smaller size.

2. Do have a look at the bra situation. One of the most joyous moments of my (India's) diet life was the discovery that I could once again buy little frippery bras made of gingham or pink lace, after a longer-than-seemly period of wearing – for want of something better – unappealing numbers with thick straps and sturdy hooks. The Russ Meyer-style bosoms, which I'd thought were there for life, did shrink, and quite dramatically too – by three cup sizes. I didn't need breast reduction surgery: I needed to lose weight. So it may be time for you to go and get measured again, and start cackling dementedly with joy in the changing room. As we're always saying, a well-fitting bra can take pounds off you and dramatically alter your shape.

Neris's journal entry:

I just had my bra fitted. It was free. It is free to get done anywhere. I'm totally and utterly blown away. I'm halfway through my diet and this is the most dramatic thing that has happened to me. I've got big boobs. I've been wearing a 40 F. Since losing the 2.5 stone I have lost my extra pair of boobs which used to sit at the top of my bra.

Anyway, picture the scene. I'm in the changing room waiting for the lady to come to see me, feeling slightly embarrassed as I don't 'do' changing rooms generally and feeling like I know everyone bangs on about getting bras fitted but I'm sure it won't make much of a difference to me. My boobs just aren't pert so they do just look like this.

The lady comes in and gasps. I always have my bra strap quite high up my back. I just thought that was just the way it was with big boobs. 'Oh, my dear . . . you must have terrible back ache.' Yes, I do. I presume I'm wearing a size too small as usual in my life. But I'm totally blown away when she measures me and says I'm not forty inches around the chest but thirty to thirty-two. And even more when she tells me I'm not an F, I'm a J or a JJ . . . I can't help but laugh. I'm Jordan but with loose skin not implants.

Oh, my god.

She puts on the right size bra for me and I can't tell you the difference it makes.

I feel like crying. I'm pert. I'm separated. I'm firm. I see my tummy for the first time since puberty. It is under what was my boob shelf and is now my enormous but under control pert boobs. I immediately look much slimmer. Much curvier. I bought two bras in the sale. Amazing. Unbelievable.

You have to get it done. Please go and get it done.

3. It's not a good idea to spend too much on new clothes, since this weight loss is an on-going project – but on the other hand your old clothes should be hanging off you by now. This is probably the perfect time for a raid on a cheap shop – buy a couple of season-appropriate outfits and rejoice! rejoice! rejoice! at the way they fit you. Don't go mad: the best is yet to come, and you'll only have to give the clothes you buy now to Oxfam. Learn to clothes-shop cheaply. Topshop became India's best friend at this stage. Primark was Neris's, although she never forgot M&S.

4. Revisit the makeup situation. We did, and it was great. Here is one of Neris's early journal entries.

Stuck to it all day but felt sad. I think it only needs one thing to set you off. Felt better after emailing India. But basically, it's because I'm going out tonight. I have nothing to wear. I feel like a loser. Am going to an awards thing with my husband and I don't feel like he is going to be proud of me.

Writing this a few hours later. I decided to make a real effort getting ready. Spent more time than I have in years doing my makeup. I really decided to put myself first and act confident. So I put on my heels which I hardly ever wear any more because they are so uncomfortable, and put on some red lipstick. The evening went well. And I stuck to the diet. Except for four glasses of wine.

5. Don't neglect your hair. A slimmer face needs a better cut. We revere our hairdressers. If you want to wait until all the weight's gone, then at least go for a trim and learn how to execute a decent, professional blow-dry.

▸ Towel-dry your hair.
▸ Most important bit: section your hair with clips, making six sections at least, with three each side of your head.
▸ Blow dry each section, pulling down your hair with a brush.

6. Establish what your best bit is. We very much liked the appearance of our collarbones, and went necklace-crazy, but you may be seriously into your legs, or arms, or face (more makeup). Once again, don't make the mistake of wandering around in minute clothing because you were a size twenty-four and are now an eighteen. Yes, it feels fabulous. And yes, you do look great. But hold your horses, and, for the time being, concentrate on accentuating one area you are especially pleased with; ideally not the upper thigh.

7. Consider heels. In the past, they may have struck you as seriously uncomfortable. Things should have lightened up by now. And there isn't a leg in the world that doesn't benefit from a bit of a heel. Even if they do make you look like a drag queen (India in modestly high heels is 6'2"). Speaking of shoes: we dropped a shoe size, so try everything on instead of blithely buying your normal size, and bear this possible reduction in mind if you shoe-shop online.

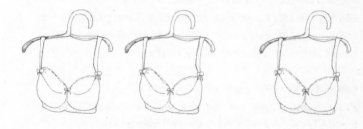

Phase Two Week Four

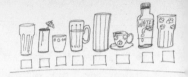

Hiya. Continue with the usual routine this week: water, supplements, breakfast, walk. Weigh and measure yourself.

Extra Vegetables

We hope you're feeling great and that you're enjoying the wider variety of foods you're no longer forbidden. This week we're upping the quantities of vegetables you're allowed. Not wildly thrilling, no, but it does help with variety cooking-wise. Up until now, we have encouraged you to eat up your greens; and to use, say, onions and tomatoes in moderation – where a recipe calls for a little of it. From now on, you can eat them more freely. We still urge you to keep at it with the green leafy veg: they're the lowest in carbs, and the best for you. But if you now want a couple of stuffed tomatoes for lunch, go right ahead. You still need to avoid potatoes – carb-city – altogether. Carrots are very carby also, but from now on you could, for instance, add a couple to minestrone – just don't eat three bowlfuls of carrot purée. Sweetcorn remains problematic, but you could certainly add a spoonful to your tuna mayonnaise. Treat peas, also very carby, as you do carrots: a handful here and there shouldn't be a problem, but more than that might be.

Coconut Milk

From this week, you can also cook with coconut milk – especially useful if you like fragrant vegetable curries, or Thai food.

Socializing and Sinning Sensibly

This week we're going to look at socializing. As we keep saying until we are blue in the face, this is a sociable diet. The foods you are eating are not what are traditionally considered diet foods, which is good news a: because you can diet on the sly if that's the way you like it, and b: because it exempts you from having to stand around at parties not being able to eat anything.

You should have worked all of this out for yourself by now, but here's a handy guide just in case. Some parties are more diet-friendly than others, and what we're going to do now is teach you how to sin sensibly if you're forced to go off-piste for one night.

The Drinks Party

Usually pretty straightforward, unless the only things on offer are sugary cocktails and baked potatoes.

Drink: DRY white wine, champagne or red wine; you can also drink clean spirits with diet tonic or soda water. We find that following each alcoholic drink with a glass of water is helpful on all counts – one wine, one water, another wine, another water, and so on. Not only do you remain relatively sober, but the water flushes out and rehydrates your system in a useful manner.

Eat: crudités, sausages on sticks, cheese on sticks, cold meats and antipasti, mini burgers without the buns, smoked salmon, cream-cheese-based spreads, little mozzarella balls, sashimi.

If all else fails: dismantle your food. This applies to all social situations. Have the quiche but leave the pastry; have the topping of the canapé but not its bready base; pick apart the sandwich and have its filling. Admittedly this isn't going to win you any awards for poise or chic, but hey – it's better than overnight weight gain.

If you're going to break your diet: don't have the baked potatoes, or the crisps or chips, or the Twiglets. Always head for the protein, even if it's accompanied by a carb, but be intelligent about it. Sushi, for instance, is a far better thing to eat, diet-wise, than a ham roll, even though both contain a mix of protein and carbohydrate. A little bit of sushi rice will hardly impact on your weight loss at this stage (it would be disastrous in Phase One); a great stonking white roll will. If you're confused, go for the option that you instinctively consider healthiest, bearing in mind what you've read in this book, and the allowed foods that are coming up in the rest of Phase Two. A buckwheat blini topped with smoked salmon and sour cream is always going to make more sense than a chocolate éclair, because you'll eventually be allowed whole grains (like buckwheat) but not white sugar or milk chocolate.

The Children's Party

Trickier, because children's parties are usually based on sugar and other highly processed/refined foods – biscuits, cupcakes, crisps and the like.

Drink: water, tea, coffee, dry white wine, red wine, champagne. Or a triple whisky on the rocks, if you're India, who finds children's parties slightly challenging.

Eat: you shouldn't feel too much pressure to eat anything at kids' parties – the few occasions when I have nicked a crisp or two, I've been given filthy looks by the mum who organized it. At the end, when the hostess is trying to palm off the leftovers on the other mums, that's another thing, but by then it's all so soggy or dry the temptation just doesn't exist! 'No thanks, I've eaten,' works pretty well. If you feel obliged to eat something, try the following. The insides of sandwiches. Mini sausages. Dismantled sausage rolls. Scotch eggs (easy on the breading). Burgers without the bun. Pizza without the base. Hummus.

If you're going to break your diet: try and do so with savoury foods rather than sweet ones. As we keep saying, sugar is your number one enemy, and as addictive as nicotine. If you absolutely have to, because it would be bad form not to, then have a sliver of birthday cake, but leave the icing. Don't have sweets, biscuits, cakes, muffins or anything similar. And drink plenty of water to help flush out all the sugar.

The Wedding

Easy-peasy.

Drink: clean spirits and mixers, dry white wine, red wine, champagne. And water. You don't want to be pissed like a mad auntie because you're not quite used to alcohol yet.

Eat: whatever's on offer: it is extremely unusual for wedding meals to be entirely carb-based. Ignore the bread basket, as usual, but have the soup, the meat or fish, the cheeses, the vegetables and salad.

If you're going to break your diet: don't. You really shouldn't have to. Weddings don't warrant it, unless you know a lot of bakers who wish to celebrate their special day by forcing three dozen different kinds of bread and pastries down your throat. There is always something you can eat at weddings, and given that you are now free to drink, the day really shouldn't be a problem.

The Funeral

Difficult, because wakes and the like are very often sandwich-based.

Drink: the usual.

Eat: what's on offer, unless you can wait until you get home.

If you're going to break your diet: well, we don't blame you. You can't go to a funeral and start picking sandwiches apart, or scraping the insides of quiches out. If you have to eat, eat, but do try to stick to the basic breaking-out rules: don't go for the highest-carb option possible on the grounds of 'If I'm going to break my diet, I'll break it in style,' and steer well clear of sugar. See below if the post-funeral event takes place in a pub.

The Dinner-Party

It ought to be entirely possible to leave out the carbs, unless your host is vegetarian and serves up a giant bowl of pasta. In which case, if it's actively rude not to, have a small helping, don't angst about it, drink tons of water and up the length of your walk tomorrow morning. NB: pasta used to make up a large part of my (India's) diet: I literally couldn't imagine living without it. Now, I find it has a really weird and slightly sinister texture – I prefer foods that require more chewing. Double NB: eat pasta – when you're allowed it again, or if you're slipping up – the way the Italians do, which is in small, starter-size quantities, not in industrial-sized horse troughs. And keep it al dente – overcooked pasta means a higher GI.

Restaurants

There is absolutely no reason to break your diet because you're at a restaurant. You could do this diet for two years and eat out three times a day, and you'd still lose all the weight you need to lose. With this way of eating, restaurants are a help rather than a hindrance. Tuck in, but stick to the rules.

The Pub/The Office Party

Pretty easy, really. You can't have crisps, but you can have salted nuts and – waah – pork scratchings, should you fancy them (we can't say we do). And you can drink the usual drinks. You can even have a kebab on the way home afterwards, sans bread. Nice.

Abroad

Very easy – really, the only country that has a catastrophic record when it comes to processed carbs and sugar is America. Happily, they also have copious quantities of meat, fish and vegetables. But be super-vigilant: nearly everything ready-made you buy from a supermarket is going to be laden with sugars, trans-fats and corn syrup. No wonder they're so blimmin' fat, frankly. They're also really big, as it were, on low-carb substitutes – low-carb meals, low-carb pasta, low-carb bread, blah di blah. Avoid these at all costs. EAT FRESH FOOD!

And when you're abroad, eat what the locals eat: tapas, not fish and chips, for instance.

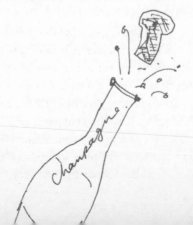

From India's journal.

On holiday. Lovely day at the beach. We took a picnic and I stupidly forgot to pack anything for myself, so then was starving. Must remember to plan. Managed to score some nuts at the beach shop. Had a latte with normal milk and vanilla syrup – thought, ah, why not. Had to swap it for normal latte. Vanilla syrup nauseatingly sweet – literally, I spat it out. I used to have one of these every day!

We came back from the beach and R was making dinner, and suddenly I was OVERWHELMED with hunger. Really rudely said sorry, I can't wait for your food, I have to eat NOW. Which I did. then I felt great. Long lecture from B about how boring it was of me not to drink.

Christmas

Christmas is really nice, but we don't quite understand why it's become an annual binge-fest – not just on the day, but from mid-December onwards. The whole country goes completely mad, and then feels really ill and out of shape, and it's all very puzzling. As you understand by now, bingeing until you feel sick has nothing to do with celebrating anything. The party season shouldn't bother you diet-wise – see above for canapé advice. You are, of course, allowed to drink. Christmas dinner itself is not remotely problematic either – just pass on the roast potatoes and double up on the turkey and vegetables. You may have bread sauce, once a year, in moderate quantities. And if you really, really love Christmas pudding, you can have a small helping of that as well.

You'll notice that we are suggesting breaking the rules every now and then in this chapter. Are you ready to break them? Only you know the answer to that one. If you still feel anxious about things like portion control, then try to stick to the rules. But if you know that one serving of Christmas pudding/a couple of illegal canapés/a small bowl of pasta aren't going to send you into a carb frenzy and destroy your eating plan, then just use your gumption and go off-piste when you really have to.

Please note, we are not saying 'whenever' you have to, or

'when you really want to'. Rule breaking is okay every once in a while, but it is not okay done regularly. It must never last more than one meal. You must never, ever stretch it out into the next day or, God forbid, week. You would be *amazed* at how quickly the weight you've spent weeks or months shedding will come back on. Amazed, and probably suicidal. So don't even go there. Have the odd bad thing – in isolation and, crucially, with your eyes wide open. Don't stick your head in the sand and feel all panicky. Do it deliberately and with your head firmly above ground. Know that it will delay you. Ask yourself if you'd rather have on-going weight loss, or delay it for the sake of a slice of birthday cake. Make knowing choices. You're no longer a ninny who just crams food into her mouth without thinking of the consequences. Thank goodness.

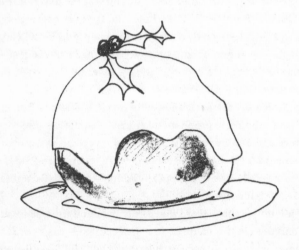

Phase Two Week Five

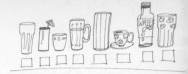

Okay – we can't put it off any longer. We're going to have to talk about exercise.

Berries

Before that, the food we are reintroducing this week is berries – all of them. Scatter them about gaily, with wild abandon: in your smoothies, on your pancakes, in sugar-free pavlovas. Have strawberries and cream – for breakfast, if you like. Speaking of which: water, supplements, breakfast, walk. Weigh and measure yourself.

Exercise

The walking should be a piece of cake by now: at the bare minimum, you've been walking every day for five weeks, though you may have been walking for months if you followed Phase One for longer than a fortnight. You will by now have dropped a considerable amount of weight. And you may be noticing that, although you can fit into clothes that are several sizes smaller, you may not be massively toned.

Here's the bummer: that particular issue is going to get worse with time, not better. The only way it's going to vanish is if you work out.

We know. That sentence sucks donkey butt. Or maybe it doesn't – maybe you're not as gym-phobic as we were. We're going to assume you are, though. Very few people with a history of fatness enjoy deporting themselves on stair machines on a daily basis.

Neris and I went down two different routes here, with similar results in the end. Unlike her I am, or was, really phobic about exercise, and thought I needed something fairly hardcore to keep me interested, plus I knew that I needed a person standing next to me forcing me to work out. So I signed up for the most brutal programme I could find: the Bodydoctor's intensive six-week course. I can't claim it was fun. I was hoping I'd become one of those people for whom exercise becomes addictive, but I didn't – although my attitude to it has changed: I now see it's a necessary pain in the arse, and that with the effort come serious rewards. The point is, the programme worked – and how. My waist shrank dramatically. Everything became harder and leaner. I dropped another half a stone. My clothes got too big again. And I suffered: remember, I hadn't exercised since school, twenty-five years before. But it worked. The basic gist is fifteen minutes of cardio on torture machines, half an hour of target-specific weights, and a further half an hour of cardio. David Marshall, aka the Bodydoctor, has a website – and dozens of celebrity endorsements – at www.bodydoctor.com. Have a look. If you despair when it comes to exercise, and want serious results, you can buy the entire programme online and do it at home. It's pared down, precise, and it gets results. And no, you won't need to buy two tons of special equipment. Neris joined a gym . . . and for the first time in her life actually went there regularly. She kept going by meeting her old friend Mari-Claire there three times a week. Mari-Claire guided Neris through the sessions and encouraged her all the way. You need a really inspiring trainer or exercise class teacher at some point just to keep you going. It is great to have someone to talk to and to spur you on and make you laugh.

Whatever you choose to do, gather information first. We're not personal trainers, and we can only tell you what worked for us. My understanding is that a minimum of three sessions of cardio is unbeatable if you want to burn fat.

Neris wrote in her diary:

My husband told me that now I've started exercising a bit, the most noticeable thing about me . . . even though I'm moving more than I've ever done before . . . is that I'm not exhausted all day every day like I used to be. Even when I was watching telly this evening I had an urge to do a deep muscle stretch . . . unheard of and strange. I didn't actually do it but I had a strong urge.

Another benefit of exercise is that it enables you to eat more

– and that it clears your conscience if you've overindulged.
It is an absolute fact that the weight comes off faster if you're
working out at the same time as dieting – but it needs to be
the right kind of workout. I know lots of quite fat people who
are marvellously supple through yoga, but they're still fat. I
know fat people who cycle every day, and they're fit – but still
fat. I know fat swimmers, and fat people who go to the gym
religiously, but stay fat. You really, really need to know what
you are doing, and what works best at shifting the weight. Our
advice would always be to go to your local reputable gym, have
a consultation, make your goals crystal-clear, and probably hire
a one-on-one trainer for a session, to ensure you're using the
equipment properly (it sounds obvious, but there is a right
and a wrong way of using those machines).

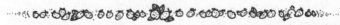

You need to bear in mind that muscle weighs more than fat,
which means that when you've been exercising for a while, your
weight may stop dipping as dramatically as it has in the past. At
this point, we suggest using a tape measure to keep track of your
changing figure – and, as always, relying on the way your clothes
fit you. As you firm up and build lean muscle, the scales may no
longer be your new best friend. The tape measure, on the other
hand, will always bring you joy.

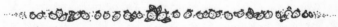

The Bodydoctor's Top Tips

Exercise as early in the day as possible, so that your metabolism
stays elevated for longer and burns more calories when you're
not exercising.

In an ideal, non-dieting world, you would eat a carb meal
before you exercise (to give you energy) and a protein meal
after exercise (to replenish lost muscle proteins). In your case,
it's fine to eat protein twice, until you get to the stage of the diet
where porridge is allowed.

Never rely on the scales, use a tape measure to chart your

progress – the tape measure never lies, scales can.

Make sure you drink plenty of water before and during exercise. If you wait until you're thirsty you're probably already dehydrated.

Make sure you warm up thoroughly. Your muscles are like an engine that needs to be the correct temperature to operate efficiently.

Concentrate on your breathing. You should always exhale on the positive movement of exercise (exertion) and inhale on the negative (return).

When you begin any exercise programme, start very gently to pre-programme your muscle memory and avoid soreness and stiffness. New exercises need to be a gentle introduction – not a blind date.

Do not concentrate on working 'harder' (quantity), but on working 'smarter' (quality). Channel all your energy positively as opposed to 'huffing and puffing', which wastes up to seventy per cent of energy expenditure.

Perform all resistance exercises slowly and smoothly. When you work quickly, momentum takes over and your muscles become the passenger instead of the driver.

Perform your cardio-vascular exercises at a moderate intensity so that you burn fat and not glycogen (blood sugar) – working at a high intensity does not burn fat.

Work with weights that exhaust you at between twenty and twenty-five reps.

Work within seventy and eighty per cent of your maximum heart rate. Any higher than this, a build-up of lactic acid will leave you very tired.

So, the time has come. This week, go and sign up for whatever form of exercise you have chosen to take. That probably means acquiring a gym membership, and going no less than three times a week. And it doesn't mean giving up on your morning walk, either. That just carries on. Don't forget to up your water once you start working out; it's very important to keep hydrated during, and after, exercise. One more point: when you start working out, it may help your energy levels to do so after a carb breakfast, i.e. after porridge. India always worked out after a pure protein breakfast, and found she still had plenty of energy, but trainers do recommend porridge. You're allowed porridge twice a week, which can be before two out of three workouts. Eat protein before the third. So you have no excuse!

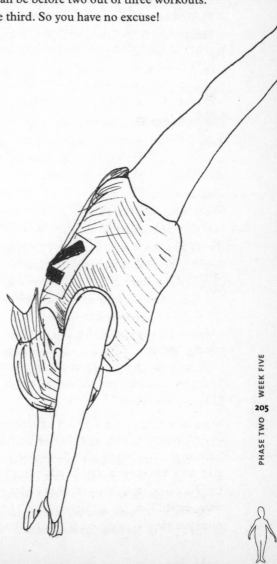

Phase Two Week Six

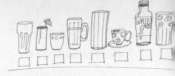

Welcome back. We hope you're not too cross with us for suggesting a gym membership. Some of you may even be enjoying going there. Even if you don't, you will not fail to notice the dramatic difference going to the gym (or whatever other proven fat-burning exercise you have committed to) makes to your body. If you still hate the gym, we sympathize. But we guarantee that you will LOVE the way it makes you look. As I (India) was saying earlier, six weeks was all it took to notice a dramatic difference.

Melons and Other Summer Fruit

This week, we are reintroducing melons, apricots, plums and peaches, which we hope for your sake are in season (bear in mind that, as a general rule, summer fruits are by and large lower in carbs than winter ones). Melon means cantaloupe or honeydew, and not watermelon, which scores very highly on the Glycaemic Index, being mostly fructose, fibre and water. Enjoy these fruits in moderation, every now and then: don't start having fruit salad three times a day. As we've already explained, all fruits have carbs and all fruits have sugars, in the form of fructose. Also bear in mind that your body is not used to fruit. Go easy. Don't have this week's fruits more than twice a week.

You know the drill: water, supplements, breakfast, walk, exercise. Weigh and measure yourself today.

This week, we'd like you to take stock.

How's the weight loss ?

As we've explained, the carbs that we've been adding over the past five weeks do slow down the process, which is why we only suggest starting Phase Two when you're within reach of your ideal weight. If you have three more stones to lose, you shouldn't be here, but still on Phase One.

However, assuming you're on this page for the right reasons, we need you to have a good long think about how you're doing.

Are you still happy at the speed with which you're losing weight? If so, all well and good – and we found the increased variety of foods we could eat compensated for the slowing down in shrinkage.

If you are not happy, though, you should be able to identify the food(s) which have caused you to slow down: if you were happily losing weight until, for instance, you reintroduced soya flour, and then suddenly nothing much happened, then you need to ask yourself whether things got moving again after a few days, or whether they're pretty much at a standstill. If they're at a standstill, then drop the soya flour until a later time. All dieters have foods that will cause them to stall; we can't tell you what yours are because we're not you. But the point of reintroducing foods slowly is for you to look out for the ones your body finds tricky.

Remember: weight loss is not linear. At this stage of the diet, it is normal – though unbelievably irritating – to plateau for a while. We define a plateau as four weeks with no weight loss or inch loss whatsoever, no matter how small, which is not caused by anything identifiable, such as eating too much chocolate or suddenly deciding to make up your own rules. There are ways out of the plateau, but first we need to establish whether you've actually hit one.

India writes in one of her diary entries:

Another half a stone down. This diet is a miracle. It has quite honestly changed my life. Am worried about Neris. She doesn't seem to be losing the amounts she would be losing if she was sticking to the diet. Which she swears she is. Hmmm. I don't know how to say it to her.

Cheating or Plateauing: a Guide

All the foods that you have reintroduced need to be eaten in moderation. Moderation does not mean 'at every meal'. Nor does it mean 'several times a day'. It means 'a couple of times a week, more if I know for sure that it doesn't affect my weight loss'. If you've been having linseed bread morning, noon and night, you are not eating it in moderation. If you've gone fruit-crazy – easily done, since our brains are hard-wired to think that fruit is good for you and that there's no such thing as having too much – then you're not eating it in moderation. (Fruit *is* good for you, but not if you're low-carbing. Then, *certain* fruits are good for you in moderation; vegetables are way better.) Ask yourself honestly whether you've sneakily been upping the quantities of these new foods to the point where you are no longer eating them moderately. If the answer is yes, STOP doing it: you may be plateauing now, but one morning soon you're going to wake up and find you've put on weight.

You still need to watch out for hidden carbs, especially in restaurant foods, prepared products (e.g. mayonnaise) and ready meals. Just because you're in Phase Two doesn't mean you can magically forget about reading the labels. Low-carbing means always being on your guard – which is why it's easiest to cook fresh foods yourself, from scratch. That way, you know exactly what's gone into them.

You really, really need to keep up with the water, now more than ever.

You can, as we've told you, go and eat a fast-food burger and leave the bun, or pick the topping off a pizza. But this is only to be done in extremis. If you find yourself lurking round the front door of McDonald's on a regular basis, you're sabotaging your diet. Don't. Make your own bacon and cheese burgers at home. That way, you'll know what's in them. And if you have a thing about fast food, you might like to scoot to the bookshop or library for a copy of *Fast Food Nation*, by Eric Schlosser. Parts of this book made India throw up.

Have you thought, 'I've got the gist of this way of eating now. What I'll do is, I'll just have some rice and a naan with my curry, and go super low-carb tomorrow and the next day'? You know what? That doesn't work. It's not going to send you running off to Fatland if you do it once in a blue moon. The problem is, lots of people do it twice a week. And then three times. And then four. And then one morning they wake up in a state of panic, wondering what's happened to the collarbones they worked so hard for.

We allow you to cheat *occasionally*, where the social situation calls for it. That doesn't mean we allow you to deliberately put yourself in that situation on a regular basis. Yes, you can have a tiny slice of cake on your daughter's birthday. But no, you can't then make a point of doing the same thing every time you pass a cake shop.

We sincerely hope that your eating is no longer emotional, and that you no longer run to the fridge when you're feeling bored, happy, upset or lonely. The thing is, we can hope all we like, but you're the only person who knows the answer to that question. Sneaking the odd chocolate finger and then eating 'by the rules' for the rest of the day is not the right thing to do. You're not plateauing, you're cheating.

Never pick and mix diets. You're eating low carb. Don't throw any other diet method into the mix, no matter how appealing or trendy it sounds. Deciding, for instance, that you're ready for the fruit-juice detox you've just read about in your Sunday supplement is going to be FATAL. Stick to one diet (this one, hopefully), and one diet only.

Never weigh or measure yourself just before or during your period. You'll get a false reading, due to water retention, among other things. If you weighed a certain amount last week and now you weigh more and your period is due, don't panic: just weigh yourself again once it's ended.

Now, if you can honestly say that none of the above applies to you, that you have been following the diet to the letter, and that nothing has happened scale or tape-measure wise for four weeks or more, then, very annoyingly, you have indeed hit a plateau. Don't be demoralized: we've all been there. Here's what to do. And, by the way, it won't work unless you've hit a genuine plateau – it's not a fast-fix for on-going cheating.

Know that this phase is surmountable. Don't despair. Don't give up. Don't think, 'the diet has stopped working'. It hasn't.

It's a phase, albeit an exasperating one, and it will pass.

Check and re-check for hidden sugars in the foods you're eating. Read every single label on every pack of food you own. If it's got sugar in it, or anything that ends in '-ose', give it away or chuck it out. Ditto anything with an unseemly number of additives. Those weird E numbers and mysterious additives stall a large number of people.

Eat more. Remember, we're eating three full meals a day, and as many snacks as it takes to keep us satisfied. If you've started skipping breakfast, or forgetting about lunch because you feel full – very easily done, since protein is so much more filling than carbohydrate, and keeps you going for longer – then please stop doing so. Skipping meals doesn't work on this diet. You must have breakfast, lunch and dinner, and as many snacks as you need in between. During a plateau, those snacks should always be a combination of protein and fat, for example cheese dipped in a creamy dressing, or smoked salmon and cream cheese wraps.

Eat more fat. Remember, this isn't a low-calorie eating plan. By this stage of the diet, now that your diet is more varied, it is easy to forget about the need to eat good fats. But you need to remember that it is the fat + protein combo that's causing the weight loss. Stick some cream and butter in your morning porridge. Don't have your steak or fish 'naked' – make a sauce.

Drink more water. Yes, even more than you're drinking already.

Cut down on coffee or tea. They stall some people.

Cut down on drink. Alcohol stimulates insulin and your body uses it – instead of your stored fat – as fuel.

Have a think about quantities. The 'free' foods you are allowed – i.e. the proteins – are free because it is almost impossible to eat them in massive quantities. But if you have been – if one fat steak isn't enough for you, and you eat three, with three lots of béarnaise, then you're going to get stalled. The 'in moderation' foods are easy to eat in excess too, especially cheese and nuts.

Up your exercise.

Still plateauing? Sure you've upped your visits to the gym?

Okay. Go back to the very beginning of Phase One for one week only, but cut out cheese and nuts. It's hardcore: it means basically eating meat, fish and eggs, plus good fats and green leafy veg and masses of water. We pretty much guarantee that this will break your stall. When you come back to Phase Two, have berries but not other fruit, and work your way up from there. The main thing to remember is that nobody plateaus for ever. There is no such thing as an eternal plateau. Sooner – we hope – or later, your weight loss will kick in again.

From Neris's journal:

My poor husband . . . his face is a picture every time I ask him if he can see a difference (in my weight). Last night he answered, 'Yeah, it's amazing how much you've lost between leaving the bathroom and getting into bed.' Maybe I'm asking him a bit too much!

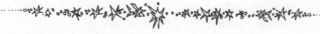

Everything all right? Revisit pages 49–50, which cover emotional eating, if you're feeling even remotely wobbly.

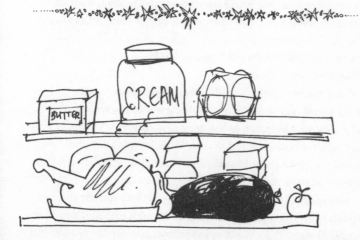

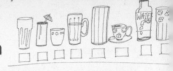

To recap: you should now be at the gym, or at the fat-burning class at the community centre, or wherever, at least three times a week. You should be drinking your water, having upped your daily intake to reflect upping your exercise. You should be taking your supplements and having a brisk morning walk. You should eat breakfast, lunch and dinner, and as many snacks as you need to keep you going in between. You should be looking pretty damned hot.

Weigh and measure yourself.

Seeds
This week we're adding seeds to the menu – that's sesame and sunflower seeds to go with the nuts you're already allowed. You can have a couple of handfuls a week. Any other seeds, such as pumpkin, are also fine.

You're nearly there, you know. You've nearly done it: another two weeks of Phase Two and you'll be eating pretty much everything.

We know we've become world-class bores on the subject of water. We're just going to do it one last time, because when we were at this stage we found that we weren't as careful about drinking water as we had been in the earlier stages of the diet.

Here's Neris's take on the subject:
Water: Your New Best Friend

Everywhere you look in all the magazines and on the telly you can't get away from somebody talking about the virtues of drinking more water. It has been going on for years now. Did people bother so obsessively about water before? Well, I don't know, but I've read it and seen it and sort of taken it in. I'd not done much about it before I started this diet.

Sometimes something as simple as drinking one more glass of water just doesn't factor into your day, does it? Also you hear people giving you so much advice that it goes in one ear and out the other.

I think I really started thinking about water when I began observing a couple of my friends who have absolutely lovely figures and are also luckily not obsessed with their weight. They really are both very fortunate. I started to notice that the one thing they have in common is that they both really knock back the water.

Take case number one: Faye, who works at a desk all day, keeps a one-and-a-half-litre bottle of water by her side and always manages to finish it by the end of the day. If she has had a late night she'll drink a bit more. When I asked her about how she keeps her Julia Roberts-like figure, she put it down completely to the amount of water she drinks. When she was younger she went to America to live and work for the summer and said that she just got out of the habit of drinking as much water as she had been. She got home again three months later and her friends couldn't believe the difference: she just looked so BLOATED and 'fat' (possibly not fat as we know it – but 'fat' comparatively speaking).

Then take case number two, my darling friend Ruth. She just sips all day, every day, and is never away from her small bottle of water. She is a mother who looks after two children all day long, and we know the stresses and strains of that, but I find it extraordinary that she has so quickly managed to regain her figure after two pregnancies in quick succession. Plus she is very, very upbeat and positive and has a ridiculous amount of energy. Again, when quizzed about her amazing physique and her healthy energy levels, she puts it down to sipping water throughout the day.

Then my hairdresser told me her golden rule for staying energetic while on her feet all day . . . loads of water. At this point, I just thought I MUST GIVE IT A GO.

I went to my local gym and they did a water level test and to my surprise they seemed shocked that I could even put one step in front of the other, because I was so dehydrated.

I went home and decided to do a mini experiment.

I wrote down my energy levels for a day when I didn't drink enough water. On that day, which was quite a hot one, I only drank two cups of decaf tea and about three glasses of water in total all day.

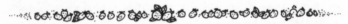

7am: Woke up feeling tired.
12pm: Not completely awake yet and slightly irritable.
3pm: Just had lunch an hour ago and now I'm ready for a sleep. Can't concentrate on the computer screen.
6pm: Okay, I'm counting the hours now till I'm home and have my feet up. Feeling irritable.
10pm: I'm loving my sofa.
Another unpleasant thing is that my urine is darkish, not clear and not much of it.

The next day I did the same experiment. Admittedly with a walk as well. And I had ten glasses of water: eight, which is what everyone should have, and two extra because I was walking. The change was ridiculous, in a good way.

7am: Woke up feeling tired (I hadn't had my water yet). Had a glass first thing. By the end of the breakfast even my husband couldn't help commenting on my 'upness' for this time of the morning.
12pm: Have been sipping through the day. Have had many a visit to the loo.
3pm: Just feel so much more energetic than I usually do. I went for a walk after lunch. I came back to my desk and genuinely felt I was more focused on what I was doing.
6pm: Okay I'm not on drugs but I just feel so energetic and happy. I've been to the loo so many times today it is extraordinary but my wee is much lighter and so much more of it. Sorry for the details.
10pm: Still loving my sofa.

I did this experiment a while ago. I'm really not exaggerating. Water works. Your mind feels more alert. You feel much more energetic. Your whole system just flushes through so much better. It sort of makes sense, if you consider that your body is made up of around two-thirds of water.

I'm a convert

I must admit I've spent a few years waking up in the morning and feeling tired before I've even got out of bed. I now drink more water and have become Miss Water-bore of the century. I feel like I have so much more energy. If you feel a bit tired, lethargic or irritable, the change you will feel is almost instant. And you'll never go back to the shrivelled, dry old days.

I now buy a small bottle of water everyday and keep it with me in my handbag and on my desk and sip it all the time, whenever I can. Then I fill it up again and keep filling it all day.

You do get a bit obsessed but I promise you, you will feel the difference.

If you are prepared to read someone who is even more obsessed about the benefits of water, try *Your Body's Many Cries for Water*, by F. Batmanghelidj.

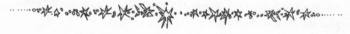

Are you a butterfly yet? Have you emerged from your cocoon? Then don't hang on to it. Chuck out – or sell – those binbags full of fat clothes.

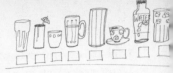

Nearly there now. Don't forget to weigh and measure yourself today.

Plain Yogurt

This week, we're reintroducing plain full-fat yogurt in moderate quantities. You may have a bowlful three times a week, which is, as I'm sure we don't need to point out, especially nice with fruit. It also means you can have raita with your curry (try adding toasted cumin seeds).

We've looked at how to get out of plateauing. This week, with the end of the 'diet' bit of this way of eating in our sights, we're going to look at how to get out of habitual cheating.

Cheating

Listen, don't feel bad. We've both done it. I (India) had some Christmas dinner one year, one thing led to another, and somehow I didn't get properly back on track for a couple of months – not because I was cheating every day, but because I'd somehow got it into my head that the odd thing occasionally wasn't going to hurt. I was right – but my understanding of 'occasionally' was wrong. It ended up meaning 'once or twice a day', more in the case of normal cow's milk in my tea. No, I didn't balloon and suddenly put on two stone. I put on half a stone, though, over those two months, and it made me very unhappy indeed. And Neris, as you've already seen from her journals, was a champion cheater for a while.

What We Have Learned About Cheating

The crucial thing about cheating is knowing you're doing it. The worst possible way of approaching the problem is to metaphorically close your eyes to it by pretending it's not happening. This is also the most fattening way.

The second crucial thing about cheating is to understand that there's always a price to pay. There is no such thing as free cheating. And you pay in pounds. That's pounds in weight, not pounds Sterling.

The third thing, bearing in mind the first two, is that, armed with this information, there is really stupid cheating and there is intelligent cheating. We say, if you're going to cheat, be clever about it.

Spontaneous cheats are the worst. They're terrible. What happens is this: you're coasting along quite happily, and you suddenly start obsessing about something or other – for the sake of argument, let's say roast potatoes. You love them. You crave them. You miss them. And everywhere you look, people seem to be eating them. It's doing your head in, but you try to push your roast potato fixation – because that's what it has become, a fixation – aside.

You don't listen to it. You ignore it. And then one weekend you're having Sunday lunch at a friend's house. You've had a couple of drinks. And there, coming out of the oven, golden and puffy and perfectly crisp, is the biggest tray of roast potatoes you've ever seen in your life. You can't stand it. You have a plateful. And then seconds. And then you feel so depressed that you think, 'Bugger it – I've completely cocked things up. I'm behaving like some mad binge-eater. Oh God. What have I done? Ah well. I'll just dunk this roast potato – my sixth – into the bread sauce, and then I'll just have some chocolate cake, and some ice cream, and another drink, and I'll think about it properly tomorrow. I'm only human. And while I'm at it, I might as well have fish and chips for supper tonight.'

The solution is this: when you are in extremis, don't push things to the back of your mind. Don't obsess about what you can't have, because that's just stupid – like spending your life in a state of abject misery because you're not Angelina Jolie and living with Brad Pitt. What's the point in moaning about that? After all, you're not thirteen years old.

But if a serious craving – one that simply won't go away – rushes to the fore, accord it the respect it deserves. Spot it coming from a distance, before it assumes mythical proportions and gets too big to manage. Say to yourself: 'Okay. Well, I *could* eat some of that. It would set me back. There would be a price to pay. But I *could* do it. I am the boss of myself. What I choose to do is up to me.' This way, you are in control – you, not the stupid roast potato.

Neris wrote in her journal one day:
Went off it today . . . got really stressed about my daughter going into hospital (which is coming up soon) and the only thing that was ever going to make me feel better was a piece of Victoria sponge cake. My favourite cake of all time. I devoured it and you know what . . . I really, really loved it, and felt better, and instead of beating myself up I just thought . . . that was lovely!

If you've somehow wandered over to this page from earlier on in the book, please go away; this doesn't apply to you yet. Now, what we would suggest at this stage of the diet is as follows: plan your cheat. Don't get to the point where you can't stand it any more and go mad with longing. If you want a roast potato, have one. Or two. Or even three. But don't allow yourself to get to the stage where you're so desperate that you have three platefuls followed by a ton of other stuff you're not allowed. Nip your craving in the bud by indulging it in a moderate way. Remain in control. Know what you're doing. Accept the consequences – and have as few carbs as possible for twenty-four hours from the next meal onwards by doing a day of Phase One.

Also, ask yourself why you are obsessing about a potato.

Another example: say it's your fortieth birthday, and a big group of you are going out for a fancy dinner. You know this is happening. You know that, just this once, you'd really, really love, on this celebratory occasion, to have anything at all you like from the menu. We say, if it's really going to enhance your life, do it. But do it cleverly. Plan ahead. Go back to Phase One for a couple of days before the event, and for a couple of days afterwards. You may put on a couple of pounds, but they'll go away again.

Whatever you do, don't just be spineless and give in to the situation. Always plan ahead. By doing so, you stay in control. And by staying in control, you always have the upper hand when it comes to your eating.

But please: once in a while only. Don't make a habit out of planned cheats. The odd one won't make much of a difference – you'll be able to manage its impact relatively easily. But if you make a habit of them and have them twice a week, your weight will go creeping back up. Not only that, but your body will become confused, and get really serious about hanging on to its fat. Which means your remaining fat will become harder and harder to shift. That's a promise.

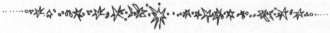

Been a while since you've had a compliment? You can't expect them all the time, and by now you should have had your fair share. If you're missing them – because people can't keep repeating themselves endlessly – then here's one from us: YOU LOOK GREAT.

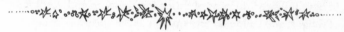

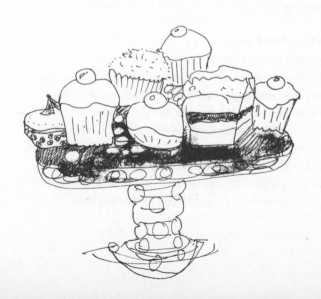

Phase Two Week Nine

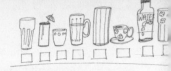

Hooray, hooray – it's the last week of Phase Two, which means you have reached the last week of the diet proper. We shower you with praise and congratulations, to say nothing of admiration. You've done a really, truly wonderful thing. Weigh and measure yourself.

Wholewheat, Stone-Ground Bread

And this week, we are reintroducing wholewheat, stone-ground bread. You may have a slice twice a week. You will need to watch yourself like a hawk during this time: not only is a slice of wholemeal, stone-ground bread (no other kind at this stage, please) very high, relatively speaking, in carbohydrates, but many, many people have a wheat allergy they don't know about. If the bread induces bloat, stop eating it.

The only thing left to say, at this late stage, is that we implore you not to give up. Obviously, you wouldn't be bonkers enough to have followed this way of eating for weeks on end, lost loads of weight, and suddenly give up. But as the variety of foods you can eat creeps up, it's quite easy to lose track of what you're ingesting, which is another, sneakier way of giving up.

Counting the Carbs

Today, therefore, we would like you to go out and buy a carbohydrate gram counter. You can get dinky little pocket ones that slip into your handbag. You don't actually need to use it very often – we both did this diet without owning one – but as the rigorous bit of the diet comes to an end, it becomes a very useful tool. What you are aiming for now is between forty and a hundred grams of carbs per day. That's still less than is contained in a bowl of super-sugary breakfast cereal, but it's enough to let you enjoy a varied and interesting diet.

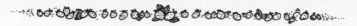

Forty and a hundred? That's a bit vague, isn't it?

It's vague in the extreme, yes. That's because we're not you. We don't know how many carbs your body can ingest without putting on weight again, or whether you're more or less likely to be at the upper or lower end of the scale.

But I don't know either!

Ah, but you do. You've been watching yourself, and will continue to do so. And that means that at some point – probably not yet, though – your weight loss will stop. You may even put on a couple of pounds. When this happens, provided you've been sticking to the diet, you know you've reached your critical point. At this stage, get out the carb counter, work out how many carbs you were eating a day before your two pesky extra pounds arrived, and stick to that number as your daily limit.

What, so now I have to start counting everything?!

No – only the new, carbier stuff. You know you lose weight by eating protein, good fats and green veg, plus the foods allowed in Phase Two – if there's a Phase Two food that stalls or bloats you, you'll have identified it and cut it out by now. Therefore, you will know at this current moment in time that you are not eating anything that throws you off course. That may change in Phase Three, when you are offered even more variety. So we're just saying, be prepared. Know what's what. You could eat several racks of spare ribs and ingest fewer carbs than you would by eating one doughnut. As the diet ends and the way of eating for life begins, we think that's worth knowing – and the way to know is to buy a carb counter.

Please now spend a moment thinking about how much you've achieved. How different you look. How different you feel. How much lighter you are. How energetic you've become. Never forget these feelings. Write them down here.

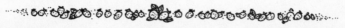

The Stakes

Neris:
- I like feeling light.
- I like having more energy. I never want to have NO energy again.
- I want to do up my size twelve trousers that I bought last week and for them not be too tight.
- I want my daughter to never remember me being frumpy and tired.

India:
- I want to continue with feeling energetic.
- I want to laugh with pleasure at fitting into a smaller size.
- I want to believe that one day my stomach will be flattish.
- I might want to get married.

What are your stakes?
Write them down here.

_____

_____

_____

_____

_____

_____

_____

_____

_____

_____

_____

_____

_____

_____

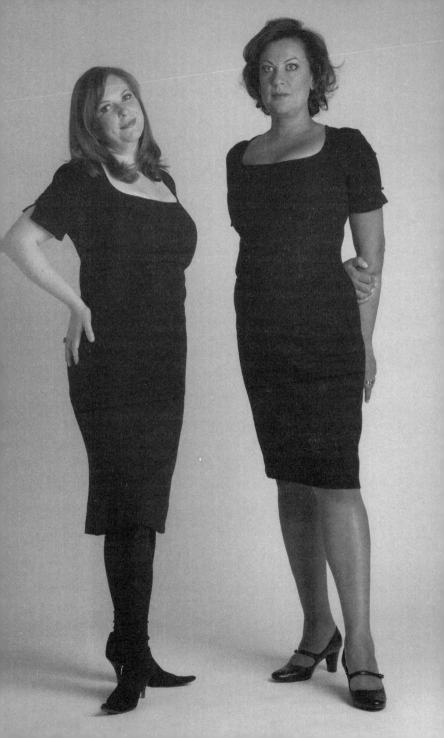

Part Four
The Diet – Phase Three

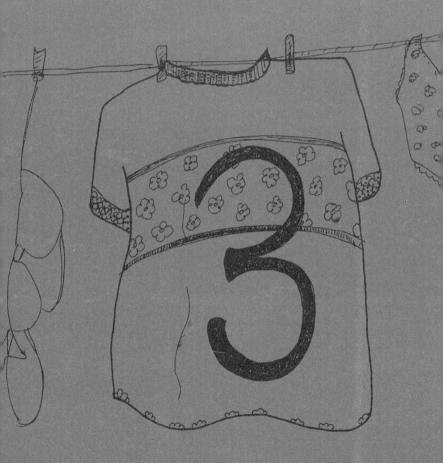

Phase Three: The Home Run

This is not a complicated diet, and from here onwards, it becomes almost absurdly simple.

What's Missing From Your Diet?
The following:

▸ Legumes, aka pulses
▸ Other fruits
▸ Starchy vegetables
▸ Whole grains (aside from the whole wheat in your occasional toast)

So they're what we're going to reintroduce next. Except that we won't be trying them out for a week or two and seeing how you do with them. We know that all of the above foods are extremely high carb, and that if you eat them on a frequent basis you'll fatten up again. There's no point in experimenting: the result is guaranteed.

So this is what we're going to do instead: not have them very often. That means once a fortnight, tops. You want lentils? You can have them, once every two weeks and in moderate quantities. You want an apple? Ditto (remember: the sweeter the fruit, the higher the fructose (sugar) content). You want a plateful of carrots? Go ahead, twice a month. Yes, it's that simple. And if you want whole grains – we're afraid white, processed grains are out as things to eat on a regular basis, though you may choose to cheat with them once in a blue moon – then do the same thing: twice a month.

That's it. And if, having consumed these things twice a month, you see no decrease in your weight loss, you may have them once a week.

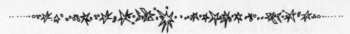

What about potatoes, bananas, sugar, pasta, white rice, white flour, biscuits, cakes and crisps?

What do you think? We don't recommend that you eat them. We have certainly eaten them during our planned cheats, but we would never in a million years make any of these foods a staple part of our diet. And we don't think you should, either.

Potatoes: nothing monstrous is going to happen if, having reached your target weight, you have the occasional potato. Let's not get phobic here. But bear in mind at all times that potatoes are ridiculously carby, and that eating too many carbs is part of what got you fat in the first place.

Bananas: rich in potassium, but then so are green leafy veg, various fish and meats, apricots, tomatoes, lettuce and parsley. But then again, the world won't collapse if you eat the occasional banana.

White sugar: this remains the crack cocaine of the food world. It does absolutely NOTHING for you except make you really fat. We say, avoid at all costs, in all of its forms.

Pasta: you can have it occasionally, say a couple of times a month, cooked al dente and served starter-size. Try to make it brown, not white.

White rice: we're not going to crap on the food that keeps half the world alive. Eat, cautiously, once or twice a month.

White flour: try to avoid (but see below). It's really not good for you, and so many people – thin people as well as fat ones – have issues with it, from IBS to bloating.

Biscuits and cakes: see white sugar. Try not to. We know you will, though – but please: there's no faster way of getting fat again than to scoff down biscuits and cakes. Not unless you have them with a side of chips, at any rate. So be ultra-aware, and if you absolutely must, have a couple once in a blue moon.

Crisps: No. Sorry. Completely pointless food. Seriously avoid. Have nuts instead.

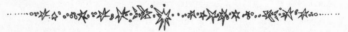

Do bear in mind that one of the many virtues of this diet is that you eat 'clean', unprocessed, additive-free food, organic where possible. The protein + fat equation is what causes the weight to come off, but eating clean food – food that hasn't been faffed around with or chemically altered or God knows what else – is also part of it. Don't ever again clog up your system with Frankenstein-like foods that make you fat and unwell, even when you've reached your target weight. Other than those, though, the world is your oyster. Eat sensibly and wisely, follow our basic rules, and fatness will be a thing of the past. If at some point in the distant future, you ever feel your weight creeping back up – though the only way this will happen is through extensive cheating – return to Phase One for a week or two. Keep working out, keep drinking your water, keep taking your supplements . . . and remember to eat and never skip meals.

Finally, we could make all sorts of claims for this way of eating. Following a low-carb regime is, according to many people, supposed to have a positive and occasionally dramatic effect on a number of complaints and conditions, from depression to polycystic ovary syndrome, and from fertility problems to general aches and pains. The anecdotal evidence is persuasive, but we're not going to go there – we're not doctors. All that we can tell you is that this way of eating worked incredibly well for us when it came to weight loss, renewed amounts of energy and general well-being. We think this is remarkable enough. If you suffer from any of the complaints above, please consult your doctor.

As the journal entries scattered throughout this book have shown, we have not always formed a united front. We went about our diets in different ways. Neris was the funny, naughty one, unable to resist the lure of the bread bin; I (India) was the boring by-the-book, square one, dutifully munching on nuts. It took Neris a while to be able to follow the diet to the letter; I did so pretty much immediately. She lied to herself (and to me) for some time; I didn't (I'm hating myself, I sound so hideously pious). I think it is fair to say that Neris's relationship with food has been indelibly marked by her dieting history, a history that stretches back a couple of decades. I don't have a dieting history. Well, I do now, obviously, but I didn't at the start of this project.

Neris really beat herself up whenever she strayed. When I went off-course, I basically felt one emotion, and one emotion only: annoyance at myself. What Neris's journals show is that her reactions were far more complex (and far more interesting) than mine: she didn't just feel annoyed but angry, sad, like a failure, hurt, out of control, panicky, despairing, pathetic, concerned about the impression she was making on her daughter; occasionally devastated. Her self-esteem plummeted dramatically every time she cheated, or even wavered; mine stayed pretty much the same. She is, I think, more self-analytical than I am, and far better attuned to the vagaries of dieting than I will ever be, but this hasn't necessarily worked in her favour: it's made her journey harder, not easier. It has also made it more impressive.

Of course, there comes a point where the diet stops being a diet and starts becoming a new way of eating – for life. I understand now, finally, that my overeating was for the greater part emotional. The way I think is not sophisticated: after I have identified a problem, I am able to sort it out and move on, without looking back. It's quite a brutal approach – Neanderthal, really. I can't really help it. I always think I'm unattractively and rather freakishly mannish for thinking and behaving this way, like some gnarled old bloke. But it does mean that, loath as I am to try to peer into the future, I don't anticipate encountering many difficulties in my eating life over the coming years. For me, overeating belongs to the past, and eating to mask an emotional issue is, well, no longer an issue for me. Being fat is over. It's not coming back if I have anything to do with it. And of course, I have everything to do with it.

I think food will continue to be more of an issue for Neris, simply because it has always been. And although I'm guessing here, I suspect that this will be true for the majority of readers of this book. If thinking about food has been a feature of your life for any length of time, if you're used to using it as both carrot and

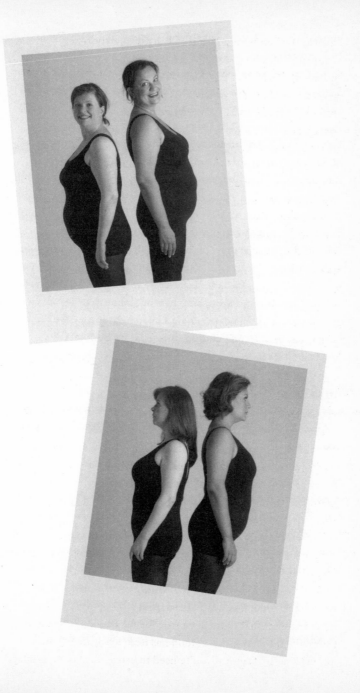

stick, you're unlikely to stop doing it overnight, despite your best intentions.

But do you know what? It doesn't matter. Because the point I am rather circuitously trying to make is that we both got there in the end. And you will, too – whether you choose to do this the hard way or the easy way; whether you come to this diet with a head stuffed full of preconceptions about calories, about carbs, about eating, and about food; or whether you come to it as a dieting virgin. Every overweight person is overweight because they eat too much of the wrong stuff. For the majority, that has less to do with greed than with a less easily identifiable hunger, a hole that needs filling, an emptiness that food somehow makes better for a while. If you are one of these people, chances are that food may continue to feature in your thoughts more often than it does in mine. Accept it. It doesn't matter. If you follow our diet, you will lose weight. And losing weight is as simple or as complicated as you want it to be. Whatever your choice, know that we did it both ways. Simple, and complicated. And we both lost five stone. You can do it too.

Here is Neris:
Losing weight has been without doubt the most difficult thing I've ever done in my life. It has been so tough. Talk about highs and lows.

I've never felt so vulnerable one week and then so strong the next. Realizing that losing weight isn't just about what you eat was a big step for me, and one I have to keep thinking about all the time. But now, I feel like for the first time I understand why I got fat. I feel like I've stopped talking to myself in such a critical way. Or at least I know when I'm doing it. I know I want to stay healthy and slim. I know it is up to me. No more excuses. What happens is completely down to me and only me. I've done it and I'm going to stick to it and nothing will stop me. And I feel so much happier.

If you ever feel yourself slipping, pick up this book again. It contains everything you need to know in order to lose weight.

That's it. We're done. Whether you've read this book all the way through before embarking on our way of eating, or whether you're done too, and have reached these final pages during your own final stages of doing our diet, thank you for reading. This diet has worked beautifully for us – it wouldn't, I don't think, be melodramatic to say it's changed our lives. We hope it changes yours, too.

And, once again: congratulations . . . for recognizing that you had a problem; for having the oomph to do something about it; for picking up this book; for following its instructions; for looking great and feeling better; for taking control. We know how hard it is. We knew you could do it. We admire you more than words can describe, and we salute you.

India Knight and *Neris Thomas.*
July 2006.

Afterword

It's now been three years since Neris and I devised, implemented and lived this diet – and we still haven't put any weight back on. Result, no? With knobs on, frankly: we're all familiar with the Slimmer of the Year scenario, whereby someone loses an incredibly impressive amount of weight, only to go back to her former shape a year or so later. That doesn't happen with this diet – not if you don't let it. We thought it might be helpful to write a little bit about how things have been for us over the past few years on the weight maintenance front.

Obviously, at first you float around on a giant pink cloud of bliss, practically levitating with happiness. You run in and out of 'normal' clothes shops, not because you need anything but for the sheer joy of being able to try stuff on, off the rail, knowing that it will fit. (Given the random sizing policy of most shops, there were even times when the item was too big. Too big! At this point, we'd practically lie on the floor, kicking our legs in the air and whooping.) We both bought a lot of new clothes in the first year after the diet – given that one of the things that had spurred us on initially was the impossibility of high-street shopping, we just couldn't resist. Here's a tip: don't just hang these new clothes in your wardrobe, but cull (or sell, or give away) anything that's too big, as and when it becomes too big. Having your old-size giant clothes lurking at the back of your closet is not helpful – they act as a sort of safety net, just in case you 'accidentally' get fat again. You're not going to get fat again, and you don't need a safety net. You're flying. You'll fly much better if you're not thinking, Oh well, I don't have to concentrate that hard, because there's a safety net down there.

Having said that, as the weeks and months go past, a degree of complacency inevitably sets in. You may have bread a couple of times a week, snaffle the odd roast potato – 'it's fine,' you tell yourself, 'it's allowed, at this stage.' And it is. But we have both found that although eating this way becomes genuinely effortless, it really pays to fight the complacency and remain vigilant at all times. A couple of times a week is fine. A couple of times a day is not. But the thing is that once you know the 'secret' of losing weight quickly and effectively, there is always a danger of thinking to yourself, 'I'll just have what I like for a couple of weeks, and go back to Phase One when I come back from my holiday. I know it works, so where's the harm?'

Now, that works beautifully if, for instance, you go camping (no, us neither – we're being hypothetical) for a fortnight and have porridge for breakfast and the odd banana as a snack. You're walking, swimming, cycling or whatever (sobbing in the rain, demanding a hotel, possibly), and nothing terrible is going to happen if you should chance across a lovely tea shop and feel overcome with desire for a scone with jam and clotted cream. But if you develop a meaningful relationship with said tea-shop, and find yourself dropping in on a daily basis, you're going to have a problem. Yes, the weight will still come off later, assuming you can force yourself back into Phase One when you come home, but it's not going to fall off in the way that it did the first time around. It's going to take a considerably longer time, and during that time you're going to become demoralized, possibly to the point of panic – and possibly to the point of thinking, Ah, sod it, which, as we all know by now, is precisely the attitude that kept you fat for so long.

Also, if you've been pigging out every day, chances are that (1) you've lost track of the importance of addressing the emotional issues that made so many of us fat in the first place (nobody *needs* a daily cream tea. You're using food as a reward, and that's not good. Thin people don't obsess about scones); and (2) you're going to find it difficult to go back to thinking of food as fuel – delicious fuel, but fuel all the same – not 'a treat', not 'naughty', not 'an indulgence'.

So, watch it. Eat the wedding cake on the Saturday if you must, but drink plenty of water on the Sunday and spend a couple of days doing strict Phase One. Have the bread sauce at Christmas, but understand that there will be consequences unless you remain, as you have been, in full control of your eating. Just as you were fat for a reason – eating too much of the wrong stuff – you are now thin for a reason: being in charge of what goes into your mouth. Stop being in charge, and you stop being thin. It's as simple as that.

Having said all of that, like the Voice of Doom, one of the great joys of this diet – though we don't think of it as a diet any more, more as a way of eating – is that once you've reached your target weight, there's room for elasticity. As we were saying above, the size 20 control pants aren't going to come falling out of the sky if you go to a friend's house and eat a plate of pasta – not, at any rate, if you compensate by eating salad and fish, or whatever, the following day. But we do feel we have to reiterate one of the central messages of the book you're holding, which is that people with weight issues are also people with head issues around food. As someone who used to eat pasta three or four times a week and love it with a deep passion, India now finds a very little goes a long way – it's a texture thing, oddly, which was never a problem in the past. But she also knows that, rather like cigarette smoking, the 'just this once' thing doesn't work for the majority of people. Nicotine is addictive, but so is sugar, and so, we would say, are carbohydrates. It doesn't mean you have to cower with terror when confronted with these things, but it does mean you have to keep thinking about them, and make informed choices. We find that extra weight and a return to sluggishness isn't a price worth paying for a week-long blow-out – in fact, oddly enough, we've lost our appetites for blow-outs. They've stopped feeling like fun, and started feeling like self-harming.

Give yourself some leeway, though. We have found, over the years, that we don't mind occasionally weighing half a stone more than our ideal weight – after years of being clinically obese, seven or eight pounds don't much bother us. We have also discovered, through trial and error, that this is an amount we can both still lose rapidly if we put a bit of effort into it (we are speaking subjectively: your mileage may vary). We imagine it all has to do with how fat you were in the first place, but, like we say, we can live with that temporary extra poundage for a little while. In both our cases, it tends to come on around Christmas-time (and, last year, around Easter) – and then it comes off again. But by this stage even Neris is strict and determined, and neither of us find it difficult to slip back into serious Phase One when the need arises. If you found Phase One painful or difficult, the best way of avoiding a repeat visit is simply to forego veering off-piste. And having said that, when we say Christmas and Easter we literally mean Christmas and Easter, i.e. twice a year for a week or so. Not twice a month, or twice a week. Our diet is brilliant, but it's not magic: follow the instructions and you will remain slim, ignore them and you won't. Everything in this book is there for a reason. That reason is to get you to lose dramatic amounts of weight, and to keep it off for the rest of your life.

Some further tips:

▸ Stay creative on the cooking front. Boredom is the enemy of this diet – you have to force yourself to be inventive. Cooking yourself the same old thing, week in, week out, is going to lead to lassitude and frustration – and unnecessarily so, because there is in fact a vast amount of stuff you can eat. Check out our *Idiot-Proof Diet Cookbook*, which puts paid to the notion that low-carb diets are about meat with a side of lard. It contains recipes we have been cooking from over the past few months – for ourselves and for our families – and it's the ultimate diet boredom-buster, though we say so ourselves.
▸ You don't have to keep taking the supplements for ever – they're expensive and can feel hard to swallow (literally). If glugging down great big capsules every morning makes you feel queasy, make sure you take yours after breakfast, i.e. not on an empty stomach. By Phase Three, you can dump the supplements, though we don't think a good daily multivit does anyone any harm and India retains her faith in the magical powers of Q10.

- It is absolutely crucial to keep drinking your water. We both found that veering from the prescribed eight large glasses stalled us on the weight-loss front, and caused us to podge up disproportionately when we did eat carbs. You've got to keep everything moving and flush everything out, and the water is **crucial**. It sounds sort of ridiculous, but we both really do believe that it is part of the key to keeping the weight off.
- Don't get complacent about exercise, either. As you know from reading this book, we believe in walking. Everyone needs to get from A to B at some point, so it's not like you have to find the time to do it. Don't go back to your bad habits and think, I weigh **X** amount, everything is lovely, I'll just lie on this sofa for a couple of hours instead of walking/gymning/whatever. Exercise sucks ass, but it works. It means you can eat more of the carbier foods, with little impact. Don't give up on it.
- Watch out for breaks in routine – holidays, new jobs, relocation and so on. There is no need for any of these to throw you off course, but you need to be prepared. Go to the music festival armed with nuts and vodka, so you don't starve to death and eat the sandwiches and beer out of desperation; seek out the local fishmonger/butcher on holiday; make a point of hunting out likely places to have lunch if you have a new job.
- And watch the alcohol. We can both stick impeccably to the basic diet, but throw in too much wine and it shows up depressingly quickly on the scales. We really, really recommend sticking to 'clean' spirits, as explained on page 177. Wine is fine occasionally, but if you sit down with a book and a bottle of Merlot on a nightly basis, your double chin is going to come back. Sad, but true.

We had such different experiences of dieting when we embarked upon this enterprise: India had never done it, Neris was the world expert. As you'll know from the earlier part of this book, we both got there in very different ways – India got on with it like some weird diet-Nazi; Neris found it harder, but always picked herself up and started again. None of this mattered in the long term. We both got there in the end, and we're both still there today – 10 stone down and as happy as clams. We know you can do it, because we did – and, like we said at the beginning of the book, if we did it, so can anyone.

India Knight and Neris Thomas,
London,
July 2007

PS: For more on this, and on all aspects of the diet, from being vegetarian to being menopausal to losing weight if you have polycystic ovary syndrome, and more, please visit *www.pig2twig.co.uk*, where a wonderful community of women (and a handful of brave men) are on hand to answer all of your queries.

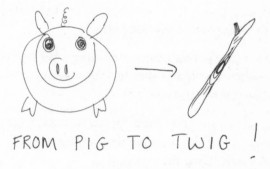

FROM PIG TO TWIG !

Inspirations

'Always bear in mind that your own resolution to succeed is more important than any one thing.' **Abraham Lincoln**

'A discovery is said to be an accident meeting a prepared mind.' **Albert von Szent-Gyorgyi**

'To follow, without halt, one aim: There's the secret of success.' **Anna Pavlova**

'If your success is not on your own terms, if it looks good to the world but does not feel good in your heart, it is not success at all.' **Anna Quindlen**

'It is possible to fail in many ways ... while to succeed is possible only in one way.' **Aristotle**

'I don't know the key to success, but the key to failure is trying to please everybody.' **Bill Cosby**

'The person who makes a success of living is the one who sees his goal steadily and aims for it unswervingly. That is dedication.' **Cecil B. DeMille**

'The man of virtue makes the difficulty to be overcome his first business, and success only a subsequent consideration.' **Confucius**

'Aim for success, not perfection. Never give up your right to be wrong, because then you will lose the ability to learn new things and move forward with your life.' **Dr David M. Burns**

'We succeed only as we identify in life, or in war, or in anything else, a single overriding objective, and make all other considerations bend to that one objective.' **Dwight D. Eisenhower**

'Success is counted sweetest by those who ne'er succeed.'
Emily Dickinson

'To freely bloom – that is my definition of success.'
Gerry Spence

'My mother drew a distinction between achievement and success. She said that "achievement is the knowledge that you have studied and worked hard and done the best that is in you. Success is being praised by others, and that's nice, too, but not as important or satisfying. Always aim for achievement and forget about success."' **Helen Hayes**

'Men are born to succeed, not fail.' **Henry David Thoreau**

'If you wish success in life, make perseverance your bosom friend, experience your wise counselor, caution your elder brother and hope your guardian genius.' **Joseph Addison**

'There's no secret about success. Did you ever know a successful man who didn't tell you about it?' **Kin Hubbard**

'Formulate and stamp indelibly on your mind a mental picture of yourself as succeeding. Hold this picture tenaciously. Never permit it to fade. Your mind will seek to develop the picture ... Do not build up obstacles in your imagination.' **Norman Vincent Peale**

'Success is not the result of spontaneous combustion. You must set yourself on fire.' **Reggie Leach**

'A minute's success pays the failure of years.'
Robert Browning

'Many of life's failures are people who did not realize
how close they were to success when they gave up.'
Thomas A. Edison

'Eighty percent of success is showing up.' **Woody Allen**

'Walking is the best possible exercise. Habituate yourself
to walk very far.' **Thomas Jefferson**

'Exercise ferments the humors, casts them into their proper
channels, throws off redundancies, and helps nature in
those secret distributions, without which the body cannot
subsist in its vigor, nor the soul act with cheerfulness.'
Joseph Addison

'Why do strong arms fatigue themselves with frivolous
dumbbells? To dig a vineyard is worthier exercise for men.'
Marcus Valerius Martialis

'All we actually have is our body and its muscles that allow
us to be under our own power.' **Allegra Kent**

'Safeguard the health both of body and soul.' **Cleobulus**

' . . . but the body is deeper than the soul and its secrets
inscrutable.' **E. M. Forster**

'I live in company with a body, a silent companion, exacting
and eternal.' **Eugene Delacroix**

'The body is an instrument, the mind its function, the
witness and reward of its operation.' **George Santayana**

'Every man is the builder of a temple called his body.'
Henry David Thoreau

'I stand in awe of my body.' **Henry David Thoreau**

'Our own physical body possesses a wisdom which we who inhabit the body lack.' **Henry Miller**

'A sound mind in a sound body is a short but full description of a happy state in this world.' **John Locke**

'He who loves the world as his body may be entrusted with the empire.' **Lao-tzu**

'There is but one temple in the universe and that is the body of man.' **Novalis**

'Choose rather to be strong of soul than strong of body.' **Pythagoras**

'If any thing is sacred the human body is sacred.' **Walt Whitman**

'Nothing has a stronger influence psychologically on their environment and especially on their children than the unlived life of the parent.' **Carl Jung**

'Act as if it were impossible to fail.' **Dorothea Brande**

'Our bodies are our gardens to which our wills are gardeners.' **William Shakespeare**

These Are a Few of Our Favourite Things

We love our products and thought you might like to hear about some of our favourites.

Hair

We both went to the same hairdresser for years without realizing. Great minds think alike when it comes to Susan Baldwin at John Frieda (020 7491 0840). She has the magic touch.

Neris uses Aveda hair products. The blow-dry lesson in the book was done at the Red Chat Chiswick Aveda salon (020 8994 3022), which is fantastic, using Aveda products. Order the products online at www.aveda.com.

We love Neal's Yard Remedies hair products. Buy online at www.nealsyardremedies.com.

We also love Bumble and Bumble Hair Powder for a quick touch-up when your hair is looking a bit 'two days ago'. Stockists 01768 891 394 and available at www.spacenk.com.

Another great hair product is Kiehl's Crème with Silk Groom. Kiehl's mail order number is 020 7240 2411.

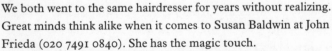

Face

Cleansers and Toners

India introduced Neris to Shu Uemura's cleansing oils and they are amazing. Take off your make-up with it as well. Shu Uemura's mail order number is 020 7240 7635.

Tesco do a fantastic beauty balm called Skin Wisdom Deep Cleansing Balm. See nearest stockist 0800 505 555.

India swears by Vaishaly's whole range of products available at Harvey Nichols nationwide (mail order 020 7235 5000, extension 2322) and direct from her clinic on 0808 144 6700 or at www.vaishaly.com.

We really love all the face products Amanda Lacey makes, especially her evening oil. They are very natural and very simple. www.amandalacey.com.

Clarins' Water Comfort One-Step Cleanser is a cleanser and a toner and is fuss-free. You don't even need water. 0800 036 3558 or www.clarins.co.uk.

Moisturizers

We love Dr Hauschka's Rose Day Cream. It is made with extract of rose petals and is really light and smells so lovely. For more details or to buy online: 01386 792 642 or www.drhauschka.co.uk.

We love Origins' Dr Andrew Weil range, especially the Mega-Mushroom Face Cream. It sounds like it is going to smell weird but is actually really lovely. 0800 731 4039 or www.origins.co.uk.

We really like Dermalogica's range of moisturizers – available in lots of salons nationwide and via www.hqhair.com.

Exfoliators

Origins' Modern Friction is great. You feel scarily clean after using it. 0800 731 4039 or www.origins.co.uk.

Clarins' Gentle Facial Peeling is absolutely brilliant. 0800 036 3558 or www.clarins.co.uk.

Eye Creams

These work:

Elemis's new Pro-Collagen Eye Renewal. 01278 727 830 or www.elemis.com.

Ren's Active 7 Radiant Eye Maintenance Serum. www.renskincare.com.

Bliss's Wrinkle Twinkle. www.blisslondon.co.uk.

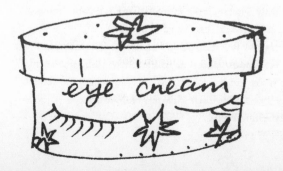

The Minimal Makeup Bag for Every Day

We struggle with anything capsule-like in our lives but there are a few makeup essentials.

Foundation

The most important thing to do is get a good foundation for smooth, even, luminous skin. A few of our favourites are below.

We worship at Laura Mercier's makeup altar. Her range includes foundations, tinted moisturizers, etc. 0870 837 7377 or www.lauramercier.com.

Prescriptives make up the colour exactly for your skin tone. No excuse for tide marks ever again! Custom-made foundation, concealer and powder available nationwide. 0870 034 2566.

Chanel's Pro Lumiére range with SPF15 is beautiful. 020 7493 3836.

Hydrotint Duo from Pixi is an amazing multi-tasking product. Tinted moisturizer with a blusher on the lid. WE LOVE PIXI. www.pixibeauty.com.

Eyebrows

Artist's Brow Stylist Mobile Essentials by Estée Lauder. This kit includes eye and brow pencils, mini tweezers, even a tube of brow gel, and is the same size as a mascara. 01730 232 566 or www.esteelauder.co.uk.

Laura Mercier also does a fantastic brow powder duo. 0870 837 7377 or www.lauramercier.com.

Mascara

Barbara Daly has created a fantastic smudge-proof mousse mascara, available at Tesco. 0800 505 555.

Of course we love Lancôme's mascaras. Their bestselling mascara is Hypnôse and it is brilliant. www.lancome.co.uk.

Sisley make great mascaras. www.sisley-cosmetics.co.uk.

Maybelline Great Lash Mascara really works. www.maybelline.co.uk.

Lipstick

Pixi Lip Booster. Put it on in the morning and it stays in place
for ages. Love it. www.pixibeauty.com.

Chanel's Rouge Allure lipsticks are fantastic. 020 7493 3836.

Estée Lauder lipsticks. We love them. Classic. 01730 232 566
or www.esteelauder.co.uk.

Lancôme's juicy tubes. Light and lovely. www.lancome.co.uk.

Body

Deodorants

We are strict about using only deodorants free from parabens
and aluminium.

We like Pit Roc at www.pitrok.co.uk, Dr Hauschka (01386 792
642) and Organic Base at www.organicbase.com.

Shower

REN's Moroccan Rose Otto Shower Wash. www.renskincare.com.

Clarins' Relax Bath and Shower Concentrate. 0800 036 3558
or www.clarins.co.uk.

www.thisworks.bathandunwind.com do fantastic shower gels.

The Art of Bathing

Scrub first:

Exotic Lime and Ginger Salt Glow Scrub by Elemis. 01278 727
830 or www.elemis.com.

Origins' Incredible Spreadable Scrub. 0800 731 4039 or www.
origins.co.uk.

Then relax in:

REN's Moroccan Rose Otto Bath oil. This is amazing. www.
renskincare.com.

You can buy the wonderful organic range Abahna online at
www.abahna.co.uk.

We really like Thalgo's Micronized Marine Algae sachets.
One hundred per cent natural and detoxing. 0800 146 041.

Body Creams

Frankincense Toning Body Cream by Neal's Yard Remedies is gorgeous. www.nealsyardremedies.com.

We really love all This Works' range, especially the Enjoy Really Rich Lotion. www.thisworks.bathandunwind.com.

Candles

Put aside that money for a takeaway and buy a candle instead.

We love, love, love Natural Magic candles because they smell incredible and they are a hundred per cent organic.
0870 460 4677 or www.naturalmagicuk.co.uk.

Rigaud from Les Senteurs. The Cyprus one is utterly amazing.
020 7730 2322.

True Grace candles are really lovely and reasonably priced.
www.truegrace.co.uk.

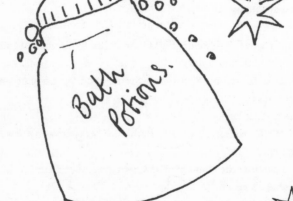
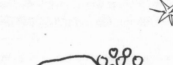

Facial Treatments

Eyes

We have a brilliant lavender eye mask made of pure organic lavender. No more mascara smudges, the lavender pouches cleverly zip in and out and the rest is fully washable. You should get a great night's sleep. www.laterre.co.uk.

Facials

Here are some of the best, for when you want to treat yourself:

All of Amanda Lacey's products. Amanda is fantastic and refreshingly down to earth. www.amandalacey.com.

The Dr Hauschka facial treatments last two hours and are amazing nationwide. 01386 792 642.

Clarins' one-hour facial makes your skin feel young again. 0800 036 3558.

Groom. Brilliant idea. One hour and two therapists. Both luxurious and efficient. 020 7499 1199.

Vaishaly's amazing facials. 0808 144 6700 or www.vaishaly.com.

Body Treatments

Elemis' body treatments rock. Find out where your nearest treatment is nationwide. 01278 727 830.

Thalgo are all sublime and fantastic. Call 0800 146 041 for your nearest treatment centre.

Other Things You Might Find Useful

Sports Bras

Whatever size you are, you should be wearing one for any amount of exercise. If you don't wear one check out www.shockabsorber. co.uk/bounceometer/shock.html. You will after seeing that.

www.boobydoo.co.uk stock every type you could ever want in any size and if they don't fit properly you can send them back. Our favourite is Shock Absorber.

Sports Clothes

Sweaty Betty have fantastic and flattering sports clothes. Order online at www.sweatyBetty.com. Neris wears her 'sweat pants' all the time.

Marks and Spencer of course do lovely stuff right up to size 24. www.marksandspencer.com.

Boots for Bigger Calves

You can look great in boots as well. In any size. Try www. duoboots.com or www.vivaladiva.com.

Tights

www.mytights.com is absolutely brilliant and has everything including Falke and Spanx. They stock not only every style of tights imaginable but also control pants. They deliver the next day.

Fitness

Here are some people we know and trust:
Mari-Claire Turley (07950 626 521 or m.c.turley@fsmail.net). The woman behind Neris's behind. Mari-Claire is fantastic, professional, fun and lovely. She will change your attitude to fitness.

Sharon Saker (07970 258 527). Seriously experienced and inspirational. Highly recommended.

India loves Tom and Paul and Grays Fitness, London NW8, 020 7483 4130.

Makeup for Special Occasions

Sarah-Jane Froom. 07725 585 476 or www.sarahjanefroom.com.

Amanda Wright made us up for this book's jacket.
amandasmakeup@aol.com.

Wardrobe Makeover

Ann Hamlyn is the stylist who gave both of our wardrobes an
overhaul. She is great. Her company is Dress Me. 020 8208 4281,
07734 870 567, www.dressme.biz or info@dressme.biz.

Journals

Don't forget to write everything down, either on a computer or
on paper. We don't care, just write.

If you're not on www.fitday.com then buy a journal at www.
paperchase.co.uk or, for an amazing journal, go to www.bookery.
co.uk and look at the 'Journalest' range. There is a journal there
specifically for health.

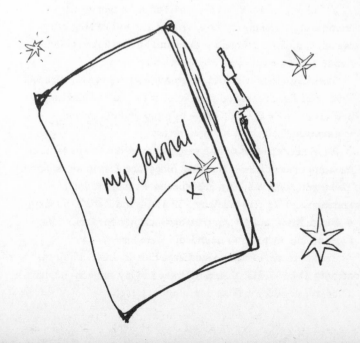

Acknowledgements

India would especially like to thank Neris, who made working on this book such a fantastic laugh from start to finish. You're a beautiful person, in every sense. Thanks also to Georgia Garrett and Juliet Annan, as ever; to my family, for the support and encouragement; to David, Tom and Paul for the excruciating but effective workouts; to Sophia Langmead for looking after my children so brilliantly – without you, there would be no books; and to Andrew for the lurve, and for finding me hot whether I'm fat, thin, or somewhere in between.

Neris wants to thank her buddy and partner-in-crime, India. Time has flown. What a laugh we've had, and what a really great friend you are.

Thanks to Juliet Annan from Fig Tree who is quite simply brilliant, and Georgia Garrett who is a fabulous agent. Thanks also to Carly Cook, Jenny Lord, John Hamilton, Tom Weldon, the lovely English rose Louise Moore, and everyone at Penguin.

Thank you so much Mari-Claire Turley for being such a great friend and getting me to move. Thanks also to The Hogarth Health Club for putting up with us and Sharon Saker, Gill Sanders and the Chiswick Pilates Practice.

Thank you to Shirley and my amazing sisters-in-law Michaela Plaice and Eve Stokes and your families for the love and support and to our lovely Emma Kirby – I simply couldn't operate without you!

A girl needs friends to lose weight. Thank you Trudie for the inspiration, Lara Turner Tomkins, Juliet Rice, Catrin Jones, Sarah Taylor and MARISA, Alison, Richenda, Samantha, and Iona and my 'forum' girls Madeleine, Charlotte and Katie T. So many thanks to Mark and Zivi, and thank God for Dixie Linder, Fay Lapaine and my rocks Jo Laurie and Ruth Joseph.

Thanks to my incredible mother, father and sister Philippa, for literally EVERYTHING and to Bruce and my gorgeous nephew Thomas as well for making our family complete.

But most of all, this is ALL for Rich. As everything is. My beautiful husband, my absolute pal and love of my life.

From us both. We both want to thank John Hamilton for your style, and everyone at Smith and Gilmour. Neris loved illustrating the book (www.nelljohnson.co.uk is her website.)

We both want to thank Shaun Webb and all at SWD for being such a big part of the book. We didn't even mind stripping off into leotards in the middle of your office. Shaun, you really are amazing. Thank you for your input, ideas and enthusiasm.

A big thank you to Sarah-Jane Froome and to Amanda Wright for making us look our best and to Ann Hamlyn for your fabulous styling; Marks and Spencer for our clothes – especially the black Magic dresses! – WE LOVE M&S. Thank you to the fabulous shop Winnie Buswell (www.winniebuswell.co.uk) for the beautiful things you sell and allowed us to borrow. Big thanks to Amy, Sonya and Tony at the brilliant Red Chat Aveda salon in Chiswick for showing us how to blow dry.

Index

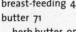

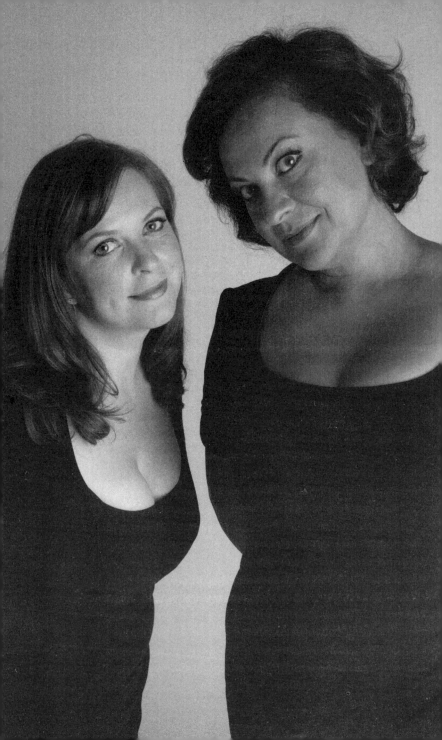